PLANT-BASED HIGH PROTEIN COOKBOOK

BODYBUILDING NUTRITION GUIDE
WITH NO MEAT RECIPES FOR ATHLETES
TO CLEAN EATING, FAT LOSS AND
MUSCLE GAINING.

Sarah Brown

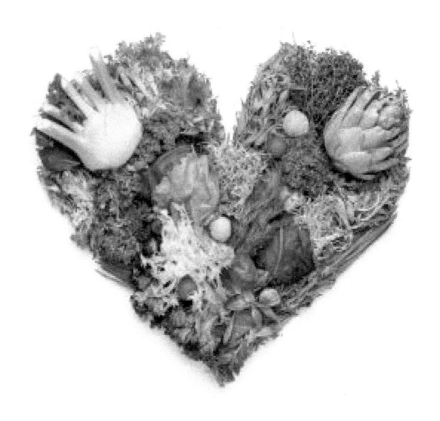

TABLE OF CONTENTS

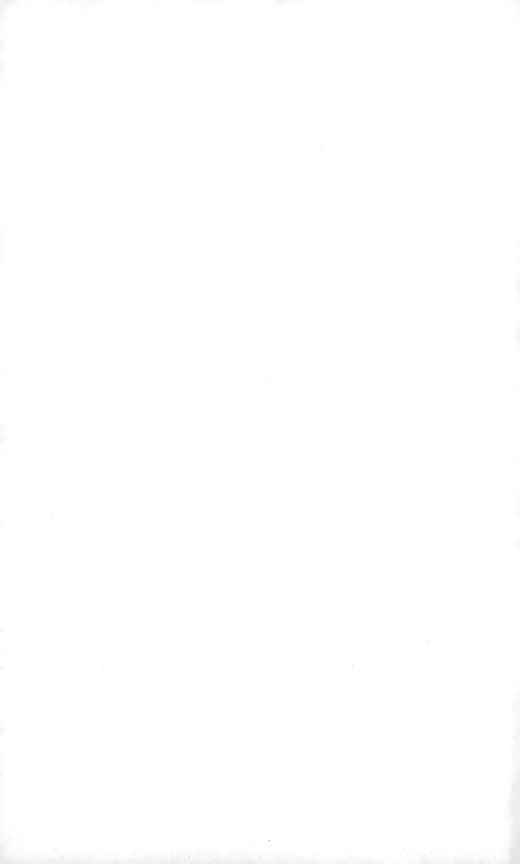

Introduction

You will be amazed by the benefits that eating whole foods can bring you. Within weeks, you may notice that you have more energy and feel greater than ever. On top of the added benefit of health, you will also be helping the environment and the animals. As you will soon be learning in the following chapters, fruits and vegetables do not need to be bland! You will be provided with dozens of delicious recipes for breakfast, lunch, and dinner.

Whether you are seasoned in the kitchen or a true beginner, this book was created for any individual who wishes to add vegan meals into their diet so that they can experience the incredible health results. All recipes that you find within this book are plant-based meals, which were created to celebrate the natural and rich flavors of your fruits and vegetables. You will find that the foods provide the nutritional value you need, which can help you fight disease and lose weight. Once you have a clear understanding of a Vegan diet, you will be learning all about high-protein foods that you will be consuming. There are many myths behind the vegan diet such as lack of nutrients and vitamins now that you will no longer be consuming animal products. The truth is nature provides us with everything we need! When you feel confident with the rules of the diet, then it is time to get to the fun action: cooking!

I hope that by the end of this book, you will be inspired to create the flavorful and protein-packed meals provided within this chapter. Each recipe is quick, easy-to-follow, and packed with the vitamins and nutrients that you need to maintain a healthy balance through breakfast, lunch, and dinner. I have assured to include a wide variety of recipes to appease even the skeptical carnivore in your life. The recipes in this book are simple to make and will inspire you to keep going. But you need not limit yourself to just these ideas. Feel free to come up with some recipes of your own. As long as you make use of the core ingredients, you can experiment to your heart's content! Let's begin!

Chapter 1: What is protein?

Healthy protein is thought to be the foundation of life, considering that it is in every cell of the body.

Healthy protein is composed of amino acids that are connected to each other in lengthy chains. There are 20 different types of amino acids, and the series in which the various amino acids are set up aids to establish the duty of that specific healthy protein.

Healthy proteins contribute to:

- Transferring particles throughout the body.
- Assisting the repair service of cells and making brand-new ones.
- Safeguarding the body from germs and infections.
- Provide appropriate development and growth in youngsters, young adults, and expectant females.

Without loading your diet plan with the proper quantities of healthy protein, you risk losing out on those crucial features. At some point, that can bring troubles, such as a loss of muscular tissue mass, that failing to expand, compromise the performance of the heart and lungs - leading to death.

One of the most shared and well-known structures in our body that rely on protein is our muscles. Muscles are attached to the bone, thus allowing us to move and function daily. While this is most obvious, the organs in our body use internal muscles to make sure that we are working and ensuring every part is doing exactly what it was intended to. Even though several parts of our body are not made of protein, they tend to be held together by protein. This includes our nervous system, organs, and blood vessels. This should show you why protein is so important in our diet.

Without a diet that contains proper protein nutrition, you would lack the components needed for tissue repair, protein to support enzymes and hormones for metabolic functions, and the aid to antibodies that help in the defense against germs and infections. While all of this may scare you away from the vegan diet or to over-consume protein, don't do this. I say this for several reasons...

For one, if you want to follow a vegan diet, I am actually going to show you that it is very possible, with all the recipes in this book! Second, if you go crazy and overload protein into your body, this can, in fact, affect your body in negative ways. Yes, there are issues if you don't have the needed amount, and yes there are issues if you take too much protein into your system. Finding the right healthy protein balance is an important thing to keep in mind when living the vegan lifestyle.

The Importance of Protein in Your Diet

Protein is a macronutrient and a very important constituent of a diet whether   you are looking to build muscle or not, as:

- It is a constituent of all body cells. As a matter of fact, nails and hair are mostly made of protein.
- Protein is required to repair and build tissue.
- Hormones, enzymes, and many other important body chemicals are made up of protein.
- It is a vital building block of cartilage, muscles, bones, skin, and blood.
- Our bodies do not stock up on protein like they do carbohydrates and fats, hence it has no reserve to draw from when the dietary requirement is not being met.

Chapter 2: Protein Requirement and How to Calculate Protein RDA Best for your Body

Healthy protein is a vital nutrient; its intake is essential for the wellness of your muscle mass and, for the wellness of the heart. Consuming healthy protein can, also, aid you handle specific illness and sustain your weight-loss initiatives. The quantity of healthy protein you need to take in is based upon your weight, exercise, age and various other variables.

Computing the RDA for protein

To figure out just how much healthy protein you ought to be consuming, there is a simple formula: take your weight, which you most likely recognize in extra pounds, and then you need to transform it to kgs. The ordinary American male evaluates to have 195.7 extra pounds (matching approximately 88.77 kilos), while the typical American woman evaluates to have 168.5 extra pounds (which amounts to a concerning 75.21 kilos).

Considering that most individuals need to consume about 0.8 grams of healthy protein per kilo of body weight, this implies that the RDA formula is:

(0.8 grams of healthy protein) x (weight in kilos).

Provided this standard, many males should consider that they should have an intake of 71 grams of healthy protein daily, due to the fact that 0.8 x 88.77 = 71.016. Ladies should eat around 60 grams of healthy protein each day, considering that the equation gives 0.8 x 75.21 = 60.168.

You can additionally simply increase your weight in extra pounds by 0.36 grams of healthy protein if you are having problem computing your body weight in kilos. This would change the RDA formula to the following:

(0.36 grams of healthy protein) x (weight in extra pounds).

There is a selection of healthy protein consumption calculators offered online if you are not comfortable in computing your RDA for healthy protein by hand. You can use sites like the "United States Department of Agriculture's Dietary Reference Intakes Calculator".

Individuals who need more protein

The RDA for healthy protein usually is 0.8 gram per kilo of body weight, lots of individuals can take in extra healthy protein safely. Professional athletes, for example, can eat as much of healthy protein as they desire as they burn a lot by exercising. Other individuals, like expecting females, nursing mothers and older generations additionally require eating even more of this nutrient.

The quantity of healthy protein you ought to eat as a professional athlete relies on the sort of exercise you take part in. Generally, individuals carrying out different workout routines ought to eat:

Minimum exercise (periodic stroll or extending): 1.0 gram of healthy protein per kilo of body weight.

Modest exercise (regular weight-lifting, quick strolling): 1.3 grams of healthy protein per kg of body weight.

Extreme training (professional athletes, routine joggers): 1.6 grams of healthy protein per kilo of body weight.

Expectant ladies, likewise, require eating even more healthy protein than the standard suggested. According to a 2016 research in the Journal of Advances in Nutrition, women need to take in between 1.2 and 1.52 grams of healthy protein per kilo of weight every day while pregnant.

The reduced quantity (1.2 grams) is appropriate for very early maternities stages of around 16 weeks, while the top quantity is advised for later maternities of about 36 weeks. The assumption of healthy protein by expectant ladies isn't just crucial for the development of the fetus; it is additionally vital in assisting the mother's body prepare to nurse their kids.

How to calculate your protein needs

It is crucial that we consume a sufficient amount of healthy protein each day to cover our body's requirements. Do you recognize just how much healthy protein you require?

Numerous professional athletes and other people that work out a lot assume that they ought to enhance their healthy protein consumption to assist them to shed their weight or construct even more muscle mass. It is real that the extra you work out, the higher your healthy protein requirement will undoubtedly be.

Healthy protein intake guidelines

Healthy proteins are the standard foundation of the body. They are comprised of amino acids and are required for the formation of muscular tissues, blood, skin, hair, nails, and the wellbeing of the interior body's organs. Besides water, healthy protein is one of the most abundant compounds in the body, and the majority of it is in the skeletal muscle mass.

Considering this, it is assuring to understand that according to the Dietary Guidelines for Americans between 2015-2020, most individuals obtain sufficient healthy protein daily. The very same record directs out that the consumption of fish and shellfish, and plant-based proteins such as seeds and nuts, are frequently lacking.

If you are an athlete, nonetheless, your healthy protein requirements might be somewhat greater considering that resistance training and endurance exercises can swiftly break down muscular tissue healthy protein.

If you are attempting to gain even more muscular tissue, you might assume that you require a lot healthier protein, yet this is not what you should do. There is proof that very strict professional athletes or exercisers might take in even more healthy protein (over 3 grams/kilograms daily), but for the typical exerciser, consumption of as much as 2 grams/per kg daily suffices for building muscle mass.

Various ways to determine protein needs

When establishing your healthy protein requirements, you can either recognize a percent of overall day-to-day calories, or you can target in detail the number of grams of healthy protein to eat each day.

Percent of daily calories

Present USDA nutritional standards recommend that adult males and females should take an amount in between 10 and 35 percent of their overall calories intake from healthy protein. To obtain your number and to track your consumption, you'll require to understand the number of calories you eat daily.

To keep a healthy and balanced weight, you need to take in about the same variety of calories that you burn daily.

Just increase that number by 10 percent and by 35 percent to obtain your variety when you understand precisely how many calories you take in daily.

As an example, a male that eats 2,000 calories each day would require to eat between 200 to 700 calories every day of healthy protein.

Healthy protein grams each day

As an option to the portion method, you can target the specific amount of healthy protein grams each day.

One straightforward method to obtain an amount of healthy protein grams daily is to equate the percent array into a particular healthy protein gram variety. The mathematical formula for this is very easy.

Each gram of healthy protein consists of 4 calories, so you will just need to split both calorie array numbers by 4.

A guy that consumes 2,000 calories daily must take in between 200 and 700 calories from healthy protein or 50 to 175 grams of healthy protein.

There are various other methods to obtain a much more specific number which might consider lean muscular tissue mass and/or exercise degree.

You can establish your fundamental healthy protein requirement as a percent of your complete day-to-day calorie consumption or as a series of healthy protein grams daily.

Healthy protein needs based on weight and activity

The ordinary adult demands a minimum of 0.8 grams of healthy protein per kg of body weight each day. One kg equates to 2.2 extra pounds, so an individual that has 165 extra pounds or 75 kg would require around 60 grams of healthy protein daily.

Healthy protein needs based on lean body mass

A new approach of finding out how much healthy protein you require is focused on the degree of the exercise (how much energy you spend) and your lean body mass. Some professionals really feel that this is an exact extra method because our lean body mass needs extra healthy protein for upkeep than fat.

Lean body mass (LBM) is merely the quantity of bodyweight that is not fat. There are various methods to identify your lean body mass, yet the most convenient is to deduct your body fat from your overall body mass.

You'll require to establish your body fat percent. There are various methods to obtain the number of your body fat consisting of screening with skin calipers, BIA ranges, or DEXA scans. You can approximate your body fat with the following calculating formula.

To determine your overall body fat in extra pounds, you will need to increase your body weight by the body fat portion. If you evaluate yourself to be 150 pounds and that your fat percent is 30, then 45 of those bodyweight pounds would certainly be fat (150 x 30% = 45).

Compute lean body mass. Merely deduct your body fat weight from your overall body weight. Utilizing the exact same instance, the lean body mass would certainly be 105 (150 - 45 = 105).

Calculating your protein needs

While the above standards offer you a general idea of where your healthy protein consumption needs to drop, determining the quantity of day-to-day healthy protein that's right for you, there is another method that can assist you in tweaking the previous results.

To identify your healthy protein requirements in grams (g), you need to initially determine your weight in kgs (kg) by separating your weight in pounds by 2.2.

Next off, choose the number of grams of healthy protein per kilo of bodyweight that is appropriate for you.

Use the reduced end of the array (0.8 g per kg) if you consider yourself to be healthy but not very active.

You should intake a more significant amount of protein (in between 1.2 and 2.0) if you are under tension, expecting, recuperating from a health problem, or if you are associated with extreme and constant weight or endurance training.

(You might require the recommendations of a physician or nutritional expert to assist you to establish this number).

Increase your weight in kg times the number of healthy protein grams per day.

For instance:

A 154 pound man that has as a routine exercising and lifting weights, but is not training at an elite degree:

154 lb/2.2 = 70 kg.

70 kg x 1.7 = 119 grams healthy protein each day.

Healthy protein as a percent of complete calories

An additional means to determine how much healthy protein you require is utilizing your everyday calorie consumption and the percentage of calories that will certainly originate from healthy protein.

Figure out exactly how many calories your body requires each day to keep your current weight.

Discover what your basal metabolic rate (BMR) is by utilizing a BMR calculator (often described as a basic power expense, or BEE, calculator).

Figure out the amount of calories you burn via day-to-day tasks and include that number to your BMR.

Next off, choose what portion of your diet plan will certainly originate from healthy protein. The percent you pick will certainly be based upon your objectives, physical fitness degree, age, type of body, and your metabolic rate. The Dietary Guidelines for Americans 2015-2020 advises that healthy protein represent something in between 10 percent and 35 percent for grownups suggested caloric intake.

Multiply that percentage by the complete variety of calories your body requires for the day to establish overall everyday calories from healthy protein.

Split that number by 4. (Quick Reference - 4 calories = 1 gram of healthy protein.)

For instance:

A 140-pound woman that eats 1800 calories each day consuming a diet plan having 20 percent of the total caloric intake consisting of healthy protein:

1800 x 0.20 = 360 calories from healthy protein.

360 calories/ 4 = 90 grams of healthy protein each day.

Compute daily protein need

To establish your day-to-day healthy protein requirement, increase your LBM by the suitable task degree.

Less active (normally non-active): increase by 0.5.

Light task (consists of strolling or horticulture): increase by 0.6.

Modest (30 mins of a modest task, thrice weekly): increase by 0.7.

Energetic (one hour of workout, 5 times regular): increase by 0.8.

Really energetic (10 to 20 hrs of regular workout): increase by 0.9.

Professional athlete (over 20 hrs of regular workout): increase by 1.0.

Based upon this approach, a 150-pound individual with an LBM of 105 would certainly need a day-to-day healthy protein amount that varies between 53 grams (if inactive) to 120 grams (if very active).

How many grams of protein should you eat per kilogram of body weight?

The quantity of healthy protein you take in is essential for your wellness. Lots of people ought to take in 0.8 grams of healthy protein per kilo of body weight, however, this quantity can alter based upon different elements. Individuals that are expecting, lactating, that have particular health and wellness problems or that are extremely energetic, commonly need even more healthy protein than the standard.

Healthy protein requirement per kilogram

You need to recognize your healthy protein demand per kg of body weight. Basically, the Recommended Dietary Allowance or RDA for healthy protein is 0.8 gram per kg of body weight.

Specific diet plans, like low-carbohydrate diet plans or the Atkins diet and even paleo diet regimens, might need you to eat even more healthy protein than this while still permitting you to take in a well-balanced diet regimen. Various other diet plans, like the Dukan diet or the predator diet regimen, concentrate on consuming only healthy protein and fat.

Raising the quantity of healthy protein you consume can be healthy and balanced and excellent, mainly if the healthy protein you are eating is originating from different resources. However, according to the Harvard Medical School, taking in even more than 2 grams of healthy protein per kg of body weight or even more can be harmful to your wellness.

According to the Centers for Disease Control, the ordinary American male values 195.7 extra pounds (or 88.77 kilos), while the typical American lady values 168.5 extra pounds (or 75.21 kilos). Given that the RDA is 0.8 grams of healthy protein for every single kilo of body weight, this indicates that a lot of males need to take in about 71 grams of healthy protein daily. Females that are a bit smaller sized ought to generally take in around 60 grams of healthy protein each day.

Chapter 3: Macros and Micronutrient

Macronutrients or macros and micronutrients or micros are molecules that the human body needs to survive, properly function and avoid getting ill. We need macros in large amounts as they are the primary nutrients for our body. There are three main macronutrients: carbohydrates, proteins, and fats. Micronutrients such as vitamins, minerals, and electrolytes are the other type of nutrients that human body requires, but in comparison to macros, micros are required in much smaller amounts.

Except for fad diets, the human body needs all three macronutrients and cutting out any of the macronutrients puts the risk of nutrient deficiencies and illness on human health.

Carbohydrates that you eat is a source of quick energy, they are transformed into glucose or commonly known as sugar and are either used right after generated or stored as glycogen for later use.

Protein is there to help with growth, injury repair, muscle formation, and protection against infections. Proteins are the compounds that are built from amino acids, which appear to be the building material for the creation of tissues in the human body. And our body needs 20 various amino acids, 9 of which cannot be produced by our body, and thus must be received from outside sources.

Dietary fat is another essential macronutrient that is responsible for many essential tasks like absorbing the fat-soluble vitamins (A, D, E and K), insulating body during cold weather, surviving long periods without food, protecting organs, supporting cell growth, and inducing hormone production.

Usually, to stay healthy, lose weight and for some other reasons we are told to count the number of calories that we intake entirely, forgetting to tell to track macronutrient intake. Calculating and monitoring macronutrient intake can help not only with making health better and reaching fitness goals but can also help you understand which types of foods improve your performance and which are bad for you. If you would like to get such a calculator, you can type in a Google search, and there you will get lots of information on the topic.

You have most likely listened to many talks about macros if you have been in the health and fitness environment for any length of time. Comprehending the truths behind macros and concerning your individual dietary needs will certainly make a difference in your very own wellness journey. In this chapter, we'll discover what macros are, exactly how to recognize if you are consuming the appropriate proportions and the very best foods for supplying them.

Macronutrients are the food classifications that give you the power to bring out our fundamental human features, and they are boiled down right into 3 groups: healthy protein, fats, and carbs. When you recognize precisely how to determine your macros, it is simple to figure out just how much calories you are placing in your body every day and just how much energy you require to burn off the extra calories.

The 3 macronutrients are carbs, fats, and healthy proteins, and they all have various duties in your body. Generally, you'll drop weight. If you desire to obtain an insight into how to monitor your macros, then keep reading.

Carbohydrates:

Composed of starches and sugars, carbohydrates are the macronutrient that your system most calls for. Your body breaks down a lot of carbs as soon as they are ingested, so they are accountable for providing you with an essential source of energy. Unless you get on a specialized consuming strategy like the ketogenic diet plan, carbohydrates ought to compose roughly 45-65% of your caloric requirements.

Carbs provide your body with sugar, its key energy source. When sugar goes into a cell, a collection of metabolic responses transforms it right into ATP (Adenosine Triphosphate), which is a kind of temporary power. Any extra sugar is changed right into a starch called glycogen, which is saved in the liver and as body fat for later usage.

Not all carbs are developed equivalent, as not all carbs are quickly absorbable or can be used for power manufacturing. Cellulose, as an example, is a non-digestible carb found in vegetables and fruits that serves as a nutritional fiber. This indicates that it aids the body get rid of waste from the big intestinal tract, subsequently maintaining it in functioning order.

Much shorter particles are much easier for your body to break down, so they are identified as basic. Complicated carbohydrates, in comparison, are bigger particles that your body takes longer to break down. Despite these distinctions, a carbohydrate is a carbohydrate in concerns to your macros.

Healthy protein:

All healthy proteins are made up of mixes of twenty various amino acids, which your body subsequently damages apart and incorporates to develop various physical structures. In other words, your body requires healthy protein to sustain the body's organ performance, power enzyme responses, and to construct your hair, nails, and various other cells.

Of the twenty amino acids, 9 are categorized as necessary, implying that your body cannot produce them, so you require to take them in via food. Those that consume a plant-based diet regimen rather than following an omnivorous diet can likewise satisfy their amino acid requirements by consuming a healthy diet plan that is composed of numerous plant-based resources of healthy protein like nuts, vegetables, and entire grains.

Like carbs, one gram of healthy protein includes 4 calories.

Fat:

Despite their destructive credibility in previous years, you should not outlaw fats from your diet plan. Your body requires fats to remain healthy and balanced, and in between 10-35% of your food needs to be composed of this macronutrient.

Fats additionally work as a power source, as it is your body's recommended approach for saving extra calories. Your system will just keep percentages of sugar in your cells, yet body fat allows you safe and secure unrestricted amounts of power rather, which you use while resting, throughout the workout, and in between meals.

When you start consuming fats, you are required to guarantee that you provide your system with fats it needs, and that cannot make itself, like omega-3 and omega-6 fats. You can find omega-3s in oily fish, eggs and walnuts, and omega-6s from a lot of veggie oils.

Water

Water makes up a considerable part of our bodies. It manages our body temperature level and helps in the metabolic process.

The Institute of Medicine suggests drinking 13 cups of water (about 3 liters) for males and 9 cups (or 2.2 liters) for females. Not sure if you are getting enough water?

Just how to figure out your macronutrient requirements

While nutritional experts advise particular proportions of each macronutrient for ideal health and wellness, every person's dietary demands will certainly be various. You can identify your specific macronutrient levels with these actions.

1. Identify your calorie requirements:

Your day-to-day calorie requirements depend on lots of variables, including your age, weight, physical fitness level, and a lot more. You can establish your degrees by tracking what you consume in an ordinary week (one in which you aren't shedding or getting weight). The ordinary degree from nowadays is an excellent indication of your calorie requirements.

2. Transform calorie counts to macronutrients

You can designate these calories in the direction of macronutrients based on the proportion you are following when you understand your calorie targets. Frequently, the macronutrient intakes varies between (AMDR) 45-65% of your day-to-day calories from carbohydrates, 20-35% from fats, and 10-35% from healthy protein.

Next off, you can identify the variety of grams to you readily available with standard mathematics. Right, here's an instance:

By thinking you require 2,000 calories daily, you can establish your fat consumption by increasing 2,000 by 0.20 (the proportion of fat for 40:40:20 macronutrient divides). That completes 400, which is the variety of daily calories to dedicate to nutritional fat. To establish your gram consumption, divide 400 by 9 (the calories in a gram of fat) for a complete need of 44 grams of fat daily.

Tips for tracking your macronutrients

Are you prepared to begin checking your macro levels? One vital action is identifying which foods will certainly aid you to achieve your goals. Eat your carbohydrates, healthy protein, and fat, so if you stick to eating those, you will make sure you are optimizing your macros.

When you initially begin checking macros, it is ideal to utilize a food range to distribute the grams amount. After you are comfortable eyeballing the quantities, you can place the food straight on your plate.

Following your body's macronutrient requirements is a clever method to remain in control of your health and wellness. The procedure of tracking grams of food could appear challenging, yet with this method, you'll acquire the abilities needed to make sure each dish is healthy enough to enhance your health and wellness.

Why do individuals count macros?

While we might be used to counting calories, a macro-focused diet plan isn't about the number of calories in your food, instead what sort of calories they are.

"To be healthy and balanced, it is crucial to obtain the best equilibrium of macros in your diet regimen," Dr. Ali states. "Sometimes individuals likewise count macros if they're attempting to drop weight, or for various other factors, such as if they're attempting to ensure they obtain the correct amount of healthy protein they require to get muscular tissue".

Locating that equilibrium suggests recognizing specifically what your body demands and what you intend to acquire or shed. It needs some computations; however, the advantages can be significant.

If It Fits Your Macros (IIFYM) diet regimen merely implies making use of a macro calculator to maintain track of the percent of healthy protein, fats, and the carbohydrates you are consuming.

Is there a fundamental macro calculator anybody can utilize?

Yes ... yet it will undoubtedly need some mathematics.

You require to figure out your basal metabolic rate or BMR. This is the rate at which your body utilizes the energy consumed and differs from one person to another. There are on the internet calculators to aid you with this, or you can do the formula on your own.

For females aged 18-30 it is: 0.0546 x (weight in kilos) + 2.33

For those aged 30-60 it is: 0.0407 x (weight in kilos) + 2.90

You can, after that, use your overall energy expense for a day.

If you are much less energetic than the basic population you increase it by 1.49 if you are at an ordinary level, you increase it by 1.63, and if you are much more energetic you increase it by 1.78

That's the amount of calories you require each day. Still with me?

From here, you can determine your macro beginning factor. Dr. Ali describes: "As a wide estimation, healthy proteins, and carbs, offer us 4 calories for each gram, and fat offers us 9 grams. If you consume a tiny smoked chicken breast, which has 6.4 g of fat and 29g of healthy protein, it would undoubtedly have 58 calories from fat and 116 calories from healthy protein - so 174 calories overall".

"We require around 50% of our calories from carbs, 15% from healthy protein, and 35% from fat, nevertheless, this obviously changes for different people".

"Regardless of whether you are attempting to slim down or construct muscular tissue, you maintain the percentages of 50% carbohydrates, 15% healthy protein, and 35% fat. You would undoubtedly transform the number of calories you would certainly have".

"If you are attempting to slim down, you require 600 calories less than your overall power expense. By doing this, you'll instantly obtain the additional healthy protein and carbohydrate you require to construct muscle mass, yet the percentages continue to be in place".

Applications such as "My Fitness Pal" which has macronutrient rankings, and "Fitocracy Macros" are complementary and can aid you to reach holds with your body's demands and count your macros.

The rationale of the macro diet regimen is that you attempt various dimensions and readjust up until you discover something that matches your needs. The diet plan does not take into account alcohol.

"A glass of rosé can have around 140 calories in it - that's more than a two-finger Ki".

Macronutrient proportions

Now that we've responded to "What are macronutrients?" we need to highlight that like diet plans and health and fitness, macronutrient proportions are not one-size-fits-all. There is no excellent macronutrient proportion that matches every person, and your demands will certainly alter according to various elements in your life.

An additional factor as to why we do not advise a really detailed macronutrient proportion is that it does not state anything regarding the high quality of the nutrients. A proportion takes into account the variety of macronutrients, which implies that carbohydrates from white sugar and quinoa are assimilated similarly.

The very best you can do is:

- Focus on equilibrium.
- Focus on whole foods.
- Enjoy your portion sizes.

Attempting to reach various macronutrient targets permits you to figure out which levels function best for you. These arrays can differ, relying on which kind of diet regimen you are adhering to. Right here are some instances of macro varieties:

Conventional diet regimen macros array:

- Healthy protein: 10-35% of calories.
- Carbohydrates: 45-65% of calories.
- Fat: 20-35% of calories.
- Low-carb diet plan macros variety:
- Healthy protein: 20-30% of calories.
- Carbohydrates: 30-40% of calories.
- Fat: 30-40% of calories.

How to calculate macros and track them

Time to place our geek cap on! A calorie is a device utilized to determine the energy-producing worth of food; however, this is not one of the most precise procedures. To get a technical explanation, a calorie is specified as the quantity of warmth needed to raise the temperature of one gram of water for one level centigrade.

Each macronutrient has a various calorie degree per gram weight.

Carb = 4 calories per gram.

Healthy protein = 4 calories per gram.

Fat = 9 calories per gram.

The overall calorie net content of food depends on the quantity of carb, healthy protein, and the fat it includes. The thinking was based on the idea that if you get rid of the greater calorie per gram macronutrient, it would certainly be less complicated to minimize the quantity of food.

Chapter 4: Diet for the 3 body types (ectomorph, mesomorph and endomorph)

There are a million and one diets on the market currently. If you can dream of it, the diet probably already exists. The vegan diet is one that has been growing in popularity for a few reasons. While some turn to veganism for ethical reasons, others consider the vegan diet for environmental purposes and even health reasons. When this diet is followed correctly, there are some wonderful health benefits that happen when you begin eating healthy. Before I get ahead of myself, let's learn what the Vegan diet is in the first place!

- An ectomorph is a typical skinny guy that have a light build with small joints and lean muscle. Usually, ectomorph's have long thin limbs with stringy muscles. Shoulders tend to be thin with little width. Ecto's need a huge amount of calories and a lot of training in order to gain weight

- a mesomorph body type tends to have a medium frame: this body type is the best for bodybuilding. These body types respond the best to weight training, but they gain fat more easily than ectomorphs.

- endomorphs have a very slow metabolism and tend to gain weight, so, they should not go overboard with carbohydrates and engage in the gym. it would be better to dissociate carbohydrates from proteins.

Different Types of Vegan

To put it in layman's terms, Veganism is about adopting a lifestyle that excludes any form of animal cruelty or exploitation. This includes any purpose, whether it be for clothing or for food. For these reasons, the Vegan diet gets rid of any animal products such as dairy, eggs, and meat. With that being said, there are several different types of vegan diets. These include:

Junk-Food Vegan Diet

A Junk-Food Vegan diet consists of mock meats, vegan desserts, fries, cheese, and heavily processed vegan foods. As you will learn later in this book, our diet avoids these foods. While technically, they are "vegan," this doesn't mean that they are good for you.

The Thrive Diet

This version of the Vegan diet is based around raw foods. The individuals who choose to follow this diet eat only whole foods that are either raw or, at the very least, cooked at very low temperatures.

Raw-till-4

The Raw-till-4 diet is just as it sounds. This diet is low-fat, where raw foods are consumed until about four at night. After four, individuals can have a fully-cooked plant-based meal for their dinner.

The Starch Solution

This version is very close to the 80/10/10 diet, which you will be learning about next. The starch solution diet follows a diet that is low-fat and high-carb. This type of vegan will focus on foods such as corn, rice, and potatoes instead of fruits.

Whole-Food Vegan Diet

This is where we come in. The Whole-Food Vegan diet is based around a wide variety of whole foods such as seeds, nuts, legumes, whole grains, vegetables, and fruits. You will find that many of the delicious recipes in this book include foods from the list above. While you may think that you will be limited when you become vegan, you will need to open your mind to all of the incredible possibilities!

What to Eat

If you are just getting started with the vegan diet, the food restrictions may come across pretty daunting. Essentially, you will be limiting your food choices to plant-based foods. Luckily, there is a very long list of foods that you will be able to eat while following this diet. Below, we will go over some of the foods that you can include on your diet—so you go into your vegan journey, full of knowledge!

Vegetables and Fruits

Obviously, fruits and vegetables are going to be very high on your list. At this point in your life, you are most likely familiar with preparing some of your favorite dishes in a certain way. It should be noted that on the vegan diet, all dairy products such as buttermilk, cream, yogurt, butter, cheese, and milk are going to be eliminated. With that being said, there are some incredible alternatives such as coconut and soy. It will take a little bit of time to adjust, but you may find that you enjoy these alternatives even more—especially because they are going to be better for your health!

There will be many vegetables you can consume on the vegan diet. It will be important for you to learn how to balance your choices so you can consume all of the nutrients you need. Within this chapter, you will be provided with a list of high-protein foods—but you will also need to consume foods such as kale, broccoli, and bok choy to help with calcium levels.

Seeds, Nuts, and Legumes

As noted earlier, protein is going to be important once you remove animal products from your diet. The good news is that legumes are a wonderful plant-based and low-fat product for vegans to get their protein. You will be eating plenty of beans such as peanuts, pinto beans, split peas, black beans, lentils, and even chickpeas. There are unlimited ways to consume these foods in a number of different dishes.

You will also be eating plenty of seeds and nuts. Both foods help provide a proper amount of protein and healthy fats when consumed in moderation. It should be noted that nuts are typically high in calories, so if you are looking to lose weight while following the vegan lifestyle, you will have to limit your portions. These foods should also be consumed without salt or sweeteners for added health benefits.

Whole Grains

Another food that will be enjoyed while following a Vegan diet is whole-grains! There are a number of products you will be able to enjoy such as wild rice, rye, quinoa, oats, millet, barley, bulgur, and brown rice! You can include these foods in any meal whether it be breakfast, lunch, or dinner! It should be noted that you will need to change how you serve some of your favorite foods. You will have to say goodbye to any animal-based products and instead, try to include more vegetables and olive oil. You can still have your morning oatmeal, but you'll have to make the switch to almond or soy milk.

Vegan Food Products and Substitutions

On the modern market, you will see a number of vegan-friendly products that have been manufactured. Some of these products include vegan mayo, whipped cream, "meat" patties, and other frozen foods. While these are great to have on hand, they are still processed foods. You will want to be careful of foods that have added sugar and salts. Any excessive additives will undo the incredible benefits the vegan diet has to offer. While, of course, they are always an option, you should try your best to stick with whole foods.

Foods to Avoid

Poultry, Meat, and Seafood

Obviously, this is a given. These foods include quail, duck, goose, turkey, chicken, wild meat, organ meat, horse, veal, pork, lamb, and beef. An easy rule you can follow is that if it has a face or a mother, leave it out. You will also have to leave out any type of fish or seafood. These include lobster, crab, mussels, calamari, scallops, squid, shrimp, anchovies, and any fish.

Dairy and Eggs

Removing dairy and eggs from a diet is typically one of the hardest parts of becoming a vegan. When you are unable to put your favorite creamer into your coffee, or simply make a batch of brownies because you have to use eggs, you will begin to notice the major difference. If you wish to become vegan, you will have to find alternatives for ice cream, cream, butter, cheese, yogurt, milk, and any type of egg.

Chapter 5: Different between animal protein and plant based protein

Perhaps you got a wise pet and determined you needed to go vegan. Perhaps you're cutting back on eating beef to enhance your ecological footprint. No matter the reason, when you lose meat into your diet, getting sufficient plant-based protein gets significant.

The Myth of the Entire Protein

To start with, it is important to be aware that it's a (quite widespread!) Fantasy Which you have to eat rice and beans together on a single plate to create complete proteins (which include all essential amino acids), such as those found in beef.

Frances Moore Lappe suggested the concept of "protein complementing" at a publication She printed from the 70s. In later versions, she adjusted the error to reflect that the prevailing scientific stance: provided that people are consuming enough calories of diverse fermented meals, they will always get all necessary amino acids and fulfill daily protein requirements. To put it Differently, rice and legumes are complementary, however you do not need to combine them together during precisely the exact same meal so as to gain from the protein every day provides by itself.

Plus, most Americans are consuming more protein than they want, so It's uncommon to become deficient (though it's much simpler without meat).

As Soon as You have Put yourself a Definite goal, write it down and Program a Listing of Actionable actions to take to achieve it. If we are adhering to the 5k instance, that may be buying new sneakers and draining out your program three times weekly to go running together with your pals. Whatever your objectives are, figuring out precisely how you are going to reach them is your first and possibly most important thing.

While it certainly is not impossible to get enough protein, zinc and B12 into your diet if you cut out all animal by products such as meat, eggs, cheese and milk, it will be a little more challenging to do so. As long as you are aware of the need to keep vegan high protein alternatives around and introduce them into your daily diet, it should all work out just fine.

Of course, one easy way to get these vitamins and minerals into your daily diet is to take a full spectrum multivitamin. There are many on the market and some are better than others. In a lot of cases, so I have been told, the liquid nutritional supplements are better than the pills because they are absorbed more easily. I don't know if that is true, talk to your doctor to make sure. Either way, introducing a quality multivitamin into your daily diet can't be a bad thing.

There are more and more vegetarian and vegan products on the market all the time. I'd bet your nearest health foods store will have a full line of vegan and vegetarian foods. Just go look around your nearest organic store and you will be amazed at your options for plant-based protein.

Along with some of the brands of organic and vegan foods you can get at your local organic store, you also have a wide variety of raw foods from which to choose. Great sources of protein are beans. All kinds of beans but especially kidney and garbanzo beans. Black beans are also loaded with protein and they can make a wild chile!

Animal-Based Ingredients

At six grams of protein and thirteen grams of fiber per thirty-five grams, chia seeds are an excellent source of protein! Chia seeds are derived from a plant that is native to Guatemala and Mexico known as the Salvia Hispanica plant. These tiny seeds also contain antioxidants, omega-3 fatty acids, magnesium, selenium, calcium, and iron! The best part is that these seeds are very versatile. While they have a bland taste alone, they absorb water fairly easy and turn into a gel-like substance. You will find later in this book; chia seeds are used in a variety of recipes from chia puddings to baked goods and even in your smoothies!

Welcome to your new favorite breakfast! Oats are a wonderful and delicious way to help get some extra protein into your diet. Half a cup of dry oats will provide you with about six grams of protein and four grams of fiber! While oats are not considered a complete protein, they have a high-quality protein, and they can be used in a number of different recipes. One of the more popular ways to include oats into your diet is to grind the oats into the flour so that you can use them for baking. Oats also include folate, phosphorus, zinc, and magnesium for added health benefits!

As a vegan, you will be saying goodbye to any dairy products. Luckily, soy milk is an excellent alternative. Soy milk is made from soybeans and is often fortified with the minerals and vitamins your body needs to thrive. On top of this, soy milk also contains seven grams of proteins per cup, vitamin B12, vitamin D, and calcium! This product can be used in a number of different baking and cooking recipes, as you will be finding out later in this book. It should be noted that B12 is not naturally occurring in soybeans, so you should try to buy a fortified variety of soy milk. With that in mind, you will also want to opt for unsweetened soy milk. This way, you will be able to keep your added sugar levels low.

Chapter 6: Breakfast

1. Peanut Butter Banana Quinoa Bowl

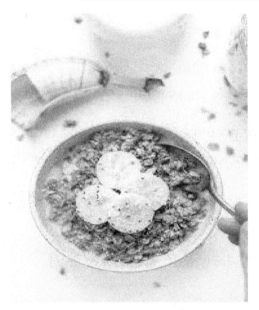

Preparation time: 15 minutes

Cooking time: 15 minutes

Servings: 1

Ingredients:

- 175ml unsweetened soy milk - 85g uncooked quinoa - ½ teaspoon Ceylon cinnamon - 10g chia seeds - 30g organic peanut butter - 30ml unsweetened almond milk - 10g raw cocoa powder - 5 drops liquid stevia - 1 small banana, peeled, sliced

Direction:

In a saucepan, bring soy milk, quinoa, and Ceylon cinnamon to a boil.

Reduce heat and simmer 15 minutes.

Remove from the heat and stir in Chia seeds. Cover the saucepan with lid and place aside for 15 minutes.

In the meantime, microwave peanut butter and almond milk for 30 seconds on high. Remove and stir until runny. Repeat the process if needed.

Stir in raw cocoa powder and Stevia.

To serve; fluff the quinoa with fork and transfer in a bowl.

Top with sliced banana.

Drizzle the quinoa with peanut butter.

Serve.

Nutrition: - Calories 718, Total Fat 29.6g - Total Carbohydrate 90.3g - Dietary Fiber 17.5g - Total Sugars 14.5g - Protein 30.4g

2. Sweet Potato slices with Fruits

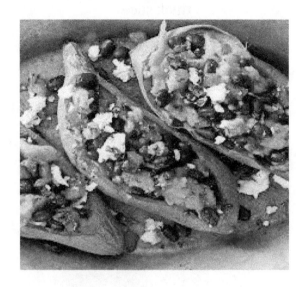

Preparation time: 10 minutes

Cooking time: 10 minutes

Servings: 2

Ingredients:

The base:

- 1 sweet potato Topping:

60g organic peanut butter

30ml pure maple syrup

4 dried apricots, sliced

30g fresh raspberries

Direction:

Peel and cut sweet potato into ½ cm thick slices.

Place the potato slices in a toaster on high for 5 minutes. Toast your sweet potatoes TWICE.

Arrange sweet potato slices onto a plate.

Spread the peanut butter over sweet potato slices.

Drizzle the maple syrup over the butter.

Top each slice with an equal amount of sliced apricots and raspberries.

Serve.

Nutrition: Calories 300, Total Fat 16.9g, Total Carbohydrate 32.1g, Dietary Fiber 6.2g, Total Sugars 17.7g, Protein 10.3g

3. Breakfast Oat Brownies

Preparation time: 10 minutes

Cooking time: 40 minutes

Servings: 10 slices (2 per serving) Ingredients:

180g old-fashioned rolled oats

80g peanut flour

30g chickpea flour

25g flax seeds meal

5g baking powder, aluminum-free

½ teaspoon baking soda

5ml vanilla paste

460ml unsweetened vanilla soy milk

80g organic applesauce

55g organic pumpkin puree

45g organic peanut butter

5ml liquid stevia extract

25g slivered almonds

Direction:

Preheat oven to 180C/350F.

Line 18 cm baking pan with parchment paper, leaving overhanging sides.

In a large bowl, combine oats, peanut flour, chickpea flour, flax seeds, baking powder, and baking soda.

In a separate bowl, whisk together vanilla paste, soy milk, applesauce. Pumpkin puree, peanut butter, and stevia.

Fold the liquid ingredients into dry ones and stir until incorporated.

Pour the batter into the prepared baking pan.

Sprinkle evenly with slivered almonds.

Bake the oat brownies for 40 minutes.

Remove from the oven and place aside to cool.

Slice and serve.

Nutrition: Calories 309, Total Fat 15.3g, Total Carbohydrate 32.2g, Dietary Fiber 9.2g, Total Sugars 9.1g, Protein 13.7g

4. Spinach Tofu Scramble with Sour Cream

Preparation time: 10 minutes

Cooking time: 15 minutes

Servings: 2

Ingredients:

Sour cream:

75g raw cashews, soaked overnight

30ml lemon juice

5g nutritional yeast

60ml water

1 good pinch salt

Tofu scramble:

15ml olive oil

1 small onion, diced

1 clove garlic, minced

400 firm tofu, pressed, crumbled

½ teaspoon ground cumin

½ teaspoon curry powder

½ teaspoon turmeric

2 tomatoes, diced

30g baby spinach

Salt, to taste

Direction:

Make the cashew sour cream; rinse and drain soaked cashews.

Place the cashews, lemon juice, nutritional yeast, water, and salt in a food processor.

Blend on high until smooth, for 5-6 minutes.

Transfer to a bowl and place aside.

Make the tofu scramble; heat olive oil in a skillet.

Add onion and cook 5 minutes over medium-high.

Add garlic, and cook stirring, for 1 minute.

Add crumbled tofu and stir to coat with oil.

Add the cumin, curry, and turmeric. Cook the tofu for 2 minutes.

Add the tomatoes and cook for 2 minutes.

Add spinach and cook, tossing until completely wilted, about 1 minute.

Transfer tofu scramble on the plate.

Top with a sour cream and serve.

Nutrition:

Calories 411, Total Fat 26.5g, Total Carbohydrate 23.1g, Dietary Fiber 5.9g, Total Sugars 6.3g, Protein 25g

5. Mexican Breakfast

Preparation time: 10 minutes

Cooking time: 10 minutes

Servings: 4

Ingredients:

170g cherry tomatoes, halved

1 small red onion, chopped

25ml lime juice

50ml olive oil

1 clove garlic, minced

1 teaspoon red chili flakes

1 teaspoon ground cumin

700g can black beans* (or cooked beans), rinsed

4 slices whole-grain bread

1 avocado, peeled, pitted

Salt, to taste

Direction:

Combine tomatoes, onion, lime juice, and 15 ml olive oil in a bowl.

Season to taste and place aside.

Heat 2 tablespoons olive oil in a skillet.

Add onion and cook 4 minutes over medium-high heat.

Add garlic and cook stirring for 1 minute.

Add red chili flakes and cumin. Cook for 30 seconds.

Add beans and cook tossing gently for 2 minutes.

Stir in ¾ of the tomato mixture and season to taste.

Remove from heat.

Slice the avocado very thinly.

Spread the beans mixture over bread slices. Top with remaining tomato and sliced avocado.

Serve.

Nutrition: Calories 476, Total Fat 21.9g, Total Carbohydrate 52.4g, Dietary Fiber 19.5g, Total Sugars 5.3g, Protein 17.1g

6. Cacao Lentil Muffins

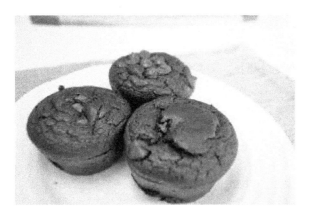

Preparation time: 10 minutes

Cooking time: 15 minutes

Servings: 12 muffins (2 per serving)

 Ingredients:

195g cooked red lentils

50ml melted coconut oil

45ml pure maple syrup

60ml unsweetened almond milk

60ml water

60g raw cocoa powder

120g whole-wheat flour

20g peanut flour

10g baking powder, aluminum-free

70g Vegan chocolate chips

Direction:

Preheat oven to 200C/400F.

Line 12-hole muffin tin with paper cases.

Place the cooked red lentils in a food blender. Blend on high until smooth.

Transfer the lentils puree into a large bowl.

Stir in coconut oil, maple syrup, almond milk, and water.

In a separate bowl, whisk cocoa powder, whole-wheat flour, peanut flour, and baking powder.

Fold in liquid ingredients and stir until just combined.

Add chocolate chips and stir until incorporated.

Divide the batter among 12 paper cases.

Tap the muffin tin gently onto the kitchen counter to remove air. Bake the muffins for 15 minutes. Cool muffins on a wire rack. Serve.

Nutrition: Calories 372, Total Fat 13.5g, Total Carbohydrate 52.7g, Dietary Fiber 12.9g, Total Sugars 13g, Protein 13.7g

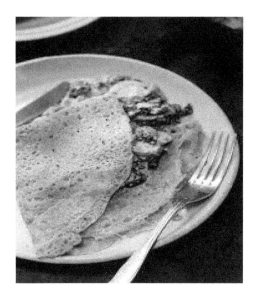

Preparation time: 20 minutes

Cooking time: 15 minutes

Servings: 4

Ingredients:

Crepes:

140g chickpea flour

30g peanut flour

5g nutritional yeast

5g curry powder

350ml water

Salt, to taste

Filling:

- 10ml olive oil - 4 portabella mushroom caps, thinly sliced - 1 onion, thinly sliced - 30g baby spinach - Salt, and pepper, to taste Vegan mayo:

60ml aquafaba

1/8 teaspoon cream of tartar

¼ teaspoon dry mustard powder

15ml lemon juice

5ml raw cider vinegar

15ml maple syrup

170ml avocado oil

Salt, to taste

Direction:

Make the mayo; combine aquafaba, cream of tartar, mustard powder. Lemon juice, cider vinegar, and maple syrup in a bowl.

Beat with a hand mixer for 30 seconds.

Set the mixer to the highest speed. Drizzle in avocado oil and beat for 10 minutes or until you have a mixture that resembles mayonnaise.

Of you want paler (in the color mayo) add more lemon juice.

Season with salt and refrigerate for 1 hour.

Make the crepes; combine chickpea flour, peanut flour, nutritional yeast, curry powder, water, and salt to taste in a food blender.

Blend until smooth.

Heat large non-stick skillet over medium-high heat. Spray the skillet with some cooking oil.

Pour ¼ cup of the batter into skillet and with a swirl motion distribute batter all over the skillet bottom.

Cook the crepe for 1 minute per side. Slide the crepe onto a plate and keep warm.

Make the filling; heat olive oil in a skillet over medium-high heat.

Add mushrooms and onion and cook for 6-8 minutes.

Add spinach and toss until wilted, for 1 minute.

Season with salt and pepper and transfer into a large bowl. Fold in prepared vegan mayo.

Spread the prepared mixture over chickpea crepes. Fold gently and serve.

Nutrition: Calories 428, Total Fat 13.3g, Total Carbohydrate 60.3g, Dietary Fiber 18.5g, Total Sugars 13.2g, Protein 22.6g

8. Goji Breakfast Bowl

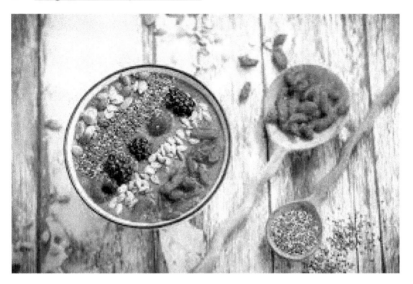

Preparation time: 10 minutes

Cooking time: 15 minutes

Servings: 2

Ingredients:

15g chia seeds

10g buckwheat

15g hemp seeds

20g Goji berries

235mml vanilla soy milk

Direction:

Combine chia, buckwheat, hemp seeds, and Goji berries in a bowl.

Heat soy milk in a saucepan until start to simmer.

Pour the milk over "cereals".

Allow the cereals to stand for 5 minutes.

Serve.

Nutrition:

Calories 339, Total Fat 14.3g, Total Carbohydrate 41.8g, Dietary Fiber 10.5g, Total Sugars 20g, Protein 13.1g

9. Breakfast Berry Parfait

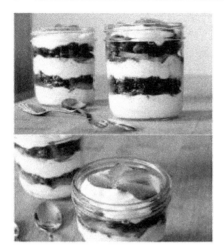

Preparation time: 10 minutes

Cooking time: 15 minutes

Servings: 1

Ingredients:

250g soy yogurt

10g wheat germ

40g raspberries

40g blackberries

30ml maple syrup

10g slivered almonds

Direction:

Pour 1/3 of soy yogurt in a parfait glass.

Top with raspberries and 1 tablespoon wheat germ.

Repeat layer with blackberries and remaining wheat germ.

Finish with soy yogurt.

Drizzle the parfait with maple syrup and sprinkle with almonds.

Serve.

Nutrition: Calories 327, Total Fat 9.4g, Total Carbohydrate 48.7g, Dietary Fiber 8.4g, Total Sugars 29.3g, Protein 15.6g

10. Mini Tofu Frittatas

Preparation time: 15 minutes

Cooking time: 25 minutes

Servings: 12 mini frittatas (3 per serving)

Ingredients:

450g firm tofu, drained

115ml soy milk

5g mild curry powder

15ml olive oil

20g chopped scallions

80g corn kernels, fresh

140g cherry tomatoes, quartered

75g baby spinach

Salt and pepper, to taste

Pesto for serving:

15g fresh basil

10g walnuts

1 clove garlic, peeled

10g lemon juice

5g nutritional yeast

20ml olive oil

30ml water

Salt, to taste

Direction:

Make the frittatas; Preheat oven to 180C/350F.

Line 12-hole mini muffin pan with paper cases.

Combine tofu, soy milk, and curry powder in a food blender. Blend until smooth.

Heat olive oil in a skillet.

Add scallions and cook 3 minutes.

Add corn and tomatoes. Cook 2 minutes.

Add spinach and cook stirring for 1 minute. Season to taste.

Stir the veggies into tofu mixture.

Divide the tofu-vegetable mixture among 12 paper cases.

Bake the frittata for 25 minutes.

In the meantime, make the pesto; combine basil, walnuts, lemon juice, and nutritional yeast in a food processor.

Process until smooth.

Add olive oil and process until smooth.

Scrape down the sides and add water. Process until creamy.

To serve; remove frittatas from the oven. Cool on a wire rack.

Remove the frittatas from the muffin tin. Top each with pesto.

Serve.

Nutrition:

Calories 220, Total Fat 14.2g, Total Carbohydrate 13.5g, Dietary Fiber 4.5g, Total Sugars 4g, Protein 15g

11. Brownie Pancakes

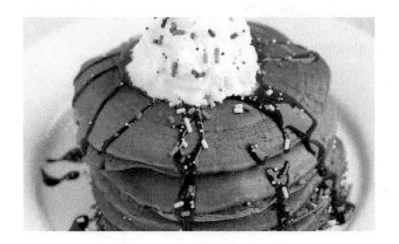

Preparation time: 10 minutes

Cooking time: 5 minutes

Servings: 2

Ingredients:

35 g cooked black beans

30g all-purpose flour

25g peanut flour

25g raw cocoa powder

5g baking powder, aluminum free

15ml pure maple sugar

60g unsweetened soy milk

35g organic applesauce

½ teaspoon vanilla paste

10g crushed almonds

Direction:

Combine cooked black beans, all-purpose flour, peanut flour, cocoa powder, and baking powder in a bowl.

In a separate bowl, whisk maple syrup, soy milk, applesauce, and vanilla.

Fold liquid ingredients into dry and whisk until smooth. You can also toss ingredients into a food blender and blend.

Heat large non-stick skillet over medium-high heat. Spray the skillet with some cooking oil.

Pour ¼ cup of batter into skillet. Sprinkle with some almonds.

Cook the pancakes on each side for 1 ½ - 2 minutes.

Serve warm, drizzled with desired syrup.

Nutrition: Calories 339, Total Fat 9.5g, Total Carbohydrate 46.8g, Dietary Fiber 11.2g, Total Sugars 6.5g, Protein 26.5g

12. Quinoa Pancake with Apricot

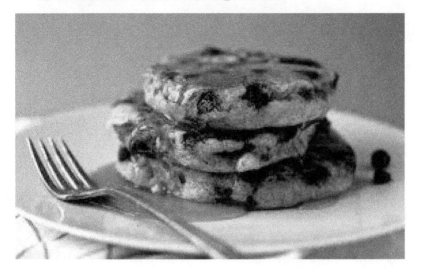

Preparation time: 10 minutes + inactive time

Cooking time: 25 minutes

Servings: 4

Ingredients:

115ml vanilla soy milk

120g apple sauce

15ml lemon juice

5g baking soda

30ml pure maple syrup

190g quinoa flour

Sauce:

60g dried apricots

5ml lemon juice

15ml maple syrup

170ml water

Direction:

Make the sauce; wash the apricots and soak in water for 1 hour.

Chop the apricots and place in a saucepan with lemon juice and maple syrup.

Cover the apricots with water and bring to a boil over medium-high heat.

Reduce heat and simmer the apricots for 12-15 minutes.

Remove from the heat and cool slightly before transfer into a food blender.

Blend the apricots until smooth. Place aside.

Make the pancakes; in a large bowl, beat soy milk, applesauce, lemon juice, and maple syrup.

Sift in quinoa flour and baking soda.

Stir until you have a smooth batter.

Heat large skillet over medium-high heat. Spray the skillet with some cooking oil.

Pour ¼ cup of the batter into skillet.

Cook the pancakes for 2 minutes per side.

Serve pancakes with apricot sauce.

Nutrition:

Calories 273, Total Fat 3g, Total Carbohydrate 51.6g, Dietary Fiber 5.2g, Total Sugars 19g, Protein 7.9g

13. Artichoke Spinach Squares

Preparation time: 10 minutes

Cooking time: 30 minutes

Servings: 8 squares, (2 per serving)

Ingredients:

340g artichoke hearts, marinated in water, drained

15ml olive oil

1 small onion, diced

1 clove garlic, minced

250g silken tofu

30ml unsweetened soy milk

40g almond meal

60g baby spinach

Salt and pepper, to taste

1/8 teaspoon dried oregano

Direction:

Preheat oven to 180C/350F.

Line 8-inch baking pan with parchment paper.

Drain artichokes and chop finely.

Heat olive oil in a skillet over medium-high heat.

Add onion and cook 4 minutes. Add garlic and cook 1 minute.

Add artichoke hearts and spinach. Cook 1 minute.

Remove from the heat and place aside to cool.

In the meantime, combine silken tofu, soy milk, salt, pepper, and oregano in a food blender.

Blend until smooth.

Stir in almond meal and artichoke mixture.

Pour the mixture into baking pan.

Bake for 25-30 minutes or until lightly browned.

Remove from the oven and cool 10 minutes.

Slice and serve.

Nutrition: Calories 183, Total Fat 10.6g

Total Carbohydrate 15.5g Dietary Fiber 6.7g

Total Sugars 3.2g, Protein 10.1g

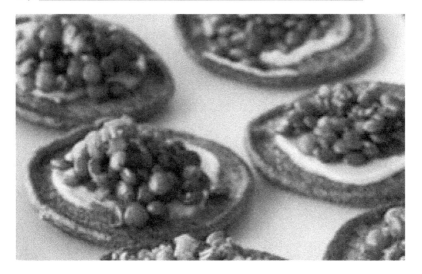

Preparation time: 15 minutes + inactive time

Cooking time: 35 minutes

Servings: 4

Ingredients:

For the blinis:

170ml unsweetened soy milk

5g instant yeast

120g buckwheat flour

75g all-purpose flour

45ml aquafaba (chickpea water)

Salt, to taste

Lentil Caviar:

15ml olive oil

1 carrot, grated

2 scallions, chopped

100g black lentils

235ml water

15ml balsamic vinegar

Salt and pepper, to taste

Direction:

Make the lentils; heat olive oil in a saucepot.

Add carrot and scallions. Cook 4 minutes over medium-high heat.

Add lentils and stir gently to coat with oil. Pour in water and bring to a boil.

Reduce heat and simmer lentils for 35 minutes or until tender.

Stir in balsamic vinegar and season to taste. Place aside.

Make the blinis; warm soy milk in a saucepan over medium heat.

In the meantime, whisk yeast with buckwheat flour, all-purpose flour, and salt to taste.

Gradually pour in warm milk until you have a smooth batter.

Beat aquafaba in a bowl until frothy. Fold the aquafaba into the batter.

Cover the batter with a clean cloth and place aside, at room temperature, for 1 hour.

Heat large skillet over medium-high heat. Coat the skillet with cooking spray.

Drop 1 tablespoon of batter into skillet. Gently distribute the batter, with a back of the spoon, just to create 2 ½ -inch circle.

Cook the blini for 1 minute per side.

Serve blinis with lentil caviar.

Garnish with some chopped coriander before serving.

Nutrition: Calories 340, Total Fat 5.9g, Total Carbohydrate 58.8g, Dietary Fiber 12.5g, Total Sugars 4.4g, Protein 14.9g

Chapter 7: Lunch

15. Cauliflower Latke

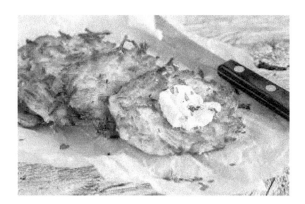

Preparation Time: 15 minutes

Cooking Time: 30 minutes

Servings: 4

Ingredients:

12 oz. cauliflower rice, cooked

1 egg, beaten

1/3 cup cornstarch

Salt and pepper to taste

¼ cup vegetable oil, divided

Chopped onion chives

Direction

Squeeze excess water from the cauliflower rice using paper towels.

Place the cauliflower rice in a bowl.

Stir in the egg and cornstarch.

Season with salt and pepper.

Pour 2 tablespoons of oil into a pan over medium heat.

Add 2 to 3 tablespoons of the cauliflower mixture into the pan.

Cook for 3 minutes per side or until golden.

Repeat until you've used up the rest of the batter.

Garnish with chopped chives.

Nutrition:

Calories: 209, Total fat: 15.2g, Saturated fat: 1.4g, Cholesterol: 47mg, Sodium: 331mg, Potassium: 21mg, Carbohydrates: 13.4g, Fiber: 1.9g, Sugar: 2g, Protein: 3.4g

16. Roasted Brussels Sprouts

Preparation Time: 30 minutes

Cooking Time: 20 minutes

Servings: 4

Ingredients:

1 lb. Brussels sprouts, sliced in half

1 shallot, chopped

1 tablespoon olive oil

Salt and pepper to taste

2 teaspoons balsamic vinegar

¼ cup pomegranate seeds

¼ cup goat cheese, crumbled

Direction:

Preheat your oven to 400 degrees F.

Coat the Brussels sprouts with oil.

Sprinkle with salt and pepper.

Transfer to a baking pan.

Roast in the oven for 20 minutes.

Drizzle with the vinegar.

Sprinkle with the seeds and cheese before serving.

Nutrition:

Calories: 117, Total fat: 5.7g, Saturated fat: 1.8g,
Cholesterol: 4mg, Sodium: 216mg, Potassium: 491mg,
Carbohydrates: 13.6g, Fiber: 4.8g, Sugar: 5g, Protein: 5.8g

Preparation Time: 10 minutes

Cooking Time: 0 minute

Servings: 6

Ingredients:

3 tablespoons lemon juice

¼ cup olive oil

Salt and pepper to taste

1 lb. Brussels sprouts, sliced thinly

¼ cup dried cranberries, chopped

½ cup pecans, toasted and chopped

½ cup Parmesan cheese, shaved

Direction

Mix the lemon juice, olive oil, salt and pepper in a bowl.

Toss the Brussels sprouts, cranberries and pecans in this mixture.

Sprinkle the Parmesan cheese on top.

Nutrition: Calories 245, Total Fat 18.9 g, Saturated Fat 9 g, Cholesterol 3 mg, Sodium 350 mg, Total Carbohydrate 15.9 g, Dietary Fiber 5 g, Protein 6.4 g, Total Sugars 10 g, Potassium 20 mg

18. Broccoli Rabe

Preparation Time: 15 minutes

Cooking Time: 15 minutes

Servings: 8

Ingredients:

2 oranges, sliced in half

1 lb. broccoli rabe

2 tablespoons sesame oil, toasted

Salt and pepper to taste

1 tablespoon sesame seeds, toasted

Direction

Pour the oil into a pan over medium heat.

Add the oranges and cook until caramelized.

Transfer to a plate. Put the broccoli in the pan and cook for 8 minutes. Squeeze the oranges to release juice in a bowl.

Stir in the oil, salt and pepper. Coat the broccoli rabe with the mixture. Sprinkle seeds on top.

Nutrition: Calories: 59, Total fat: 4.4g, Saturated fat: 0.6g, Sodium: 164mg, Potassium: 160mg, Carbohydrates: 4.1g, Fiber: 1.6g, Sugar: 2g, Protein: 2.2g

19. **Whipped Potatoes**

Preparation Time: 20 minutes

Cooking Time: 35 minutes

Servings: 10

Ingredients:

4 cups water

3 lb. potatoes, sliced into cubes

3 cloves garlic, crushed

6 tablespoons butter

2 bay leaves

10 sage leaves

½ cup Greek yogurt

¼ cup low-fat milk

Salt to taste

Direction

Boil the potatoes in water for 30 minutes or until tender.

Drain.

In a pan over medium heat, cook the garlic in butter for 1 minute.

Add the sage and cook for 5 more minutes.

Discard the garlic.

Use a fork to mash the potatoes.

Whip using an electric mixer while gradually adding the butter, yogurt, and milk.

Season with salt.

Nutrition: Calories: 169, Total fat: 7.6g, Saturated fat: 4.7g, Cholesterol: 21mg, Sodium: 251mg, Potassium: 519mg, Carbohydrates: 22.1g, Fiber: 1.5g, Sugar: 2g, Protein: 4.2g

20. Garlic Mashed Potatoes & Turnips

Preparation Time: 20 minutes

Cooking Time: 30 minutes

Servings: 8

Ingredients:

1 head garlic

1 teaspoon olive oil

1 lb. turnips, sliced into cubes

2 lb. potatoes, sliced into cubes

½ cup almond milk

½ cup Parmesan cheese, grated

1 tablespoon fresh thyme, chopped

1 tablespoon fresh chives, chopped

2 tablespoons butter

Salt and pepper to taste

Direction

Preheat your oven to 375 degrees F.

Slice the tip off the garlic head.

Drizzle with a little oil and roast in the oven for 45 minutes.

Boil the turnips and potatoes in a pot of water for 30 minutes or until tender.

Add all the ingredients to a food processor along with the garlic.

Pulse until smooth.

Nutrition: Calories: 141, Total fat: 3.2g, Saturated fat: 1.5g, Cholesterol: 7mg, Sodium: 284mg, Potassium: 676mg, Carbohydrates: 24.6g, Fiber: 3.1g, Sugar: 4g, Protein: 4.6g

21. Green Beans with Bacon

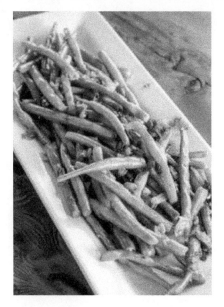

Preparation Time: 15 minutes

Cooking Time: 20 minutes

Servings: 8

Ingredients:

2 slices bacon, chopped

1 shallot, chopped

24 oz. green beans

Salt and pepper to taste

½ teaspoon smoked paprika

1 teaspoon lemon juice

2 teaspoons vinegar

Direction

Preheat your oven to 450 degrees F.

Add the bacon in the baking pan and roast for 5 minutes.

Stir in the shallot and beans.

Season with salt, pepper and paprika.

Roast for 10 minutes.

Drizzle with the lemon juice and vinegar.

Roast for another 2 minutes.

Nutrition: Calories: 49, Total fat: 1.2g, Saturated fat: 0.4g, Cholesterol: 3mg, Sodium: 192mg, Potassium: 249mg, Carbohydrates: 8.1g, Fiber: 3g, Sugar: 4g, Protein: 2.9g

22. Coconut Brussels Sprouts

Preparation Time: 15 minutes

Cooking Time: 10 minutes

Servings: 4

Ingredients:

1 lb. Brussels sprouts, trimmed and sliced in half

2 tablespoons coconut oil

¼ cup coconut water

1 tablespoon soy sauce

Direction:

In a pan over medium heat, add the coconut oil and cook the Brussels sprouts for 4 minutes.

Pour in the coconut water.

Cook for 3 minutes. Add the soy sauce and cook for another 1 minute.

Nutrition: Calories: 114, Total fat: 7.1g, Saturated fat: 5.7g

Sodium: 269mg, Potassium: 483mg, Carbohydrates: 11.1g, Fiber: 4.3g, Sugar: 3g, Protein: 4g

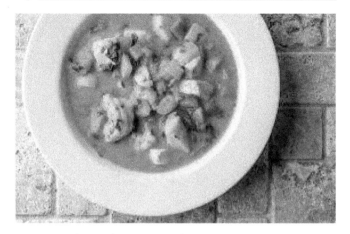

Preparation Time: 30 minutes

Cooking Time: 1 hour

Servings: 4

Ingredients:

2 cups water

¾ cup brown rice

1 tablespoon vegetable oil

1 tablespoon ginger, chopped

1 tablespoon garlic, chopped

1 sweet potato, sliced into cubes

1 bell pepper, sliced

1 tablespoon curry powder

Salt to taste

15 oz. coconut milk

4 cod fillets

2 teaspoons freshly squeezed lime juice

3 tablespoons cilantro, chopped

Direction:

Place the water and rice in a saucepan.

Bring to a boil and then simmer for 30 to 40 minutes. Set aside.

Pour the oil in a pan over medium heat.

Cook the garlic for 30 seconds.

Add the sweet potatoes and bell pepper.

Season with curry powder and salt.

Mix well. Pour in the coconut milk. Simmer for 15 minutes.

Nestle the fish into the sauce and cook for another 10 minutes.

Stir in the lime juice and cilantro.

Serve with the rice.

Nutrition: Calories: 382, Total fat: 11.3g, Saturated fat: 4.8g, Cholesterol: 45mg, Sodium: 413mg, Potassium: 736mg, Carbohydrates: 49.5g, Fiber: 5.3g, Sugar: 8g, Protein: 19.2g

24. Rice Bowl with Edamame

Preparation Time: 10 minutes

Cooking Time: 3 hours and 50 minutes

Servings: 6

Ingredients:

1 tablespoon butter, melted

¾ cup brown rice (uncooked)

1 cup wild rice (uncooked)

Cooking spray

4 cups vegetable stock

8 oz. shelled edamame

1 onion, chopped

Salt to taste

½ cup dried cherries, sliced

½ cup pecans, toasted and sliced

1 tablespoon red wine vinegar

Direction:

Add the rice and butter in a slow cooker sprayed with oil.

Pour in the stock and stir in the edamame and onions.

Season with salt.

Seal the pot.

Cook on high for 3 hours and 30 minutes.

Stir in the dried cherries. Let sit for 5 minutes.

Stir in the rest of the ingredients before serving.

Nutrition: Calories: 381, Total fat: 12g 18 %, Saturated fat: 2g

Sodium: 459mg, Carbohydrates: 61g, Fiber: 7g, Sugar: 13g, Protein: 12g.

25. Creamy Polenta

Preparation Time: 5 minutes

Cooking Time: 45 minutes

Servings: 8

Ingredients:

1 1/3 cup cornmeal

6 cups water

Salt to taste

Direction

Mix all the ingredients in a pan over medium high heat.

Boil and then simmer for 5 minutes.

Reduce the heat to low.

Stir until creamy for 45 minutes.

Let sit before serving.

Nutrition: Calories: 74, Total fat: 0.7g, Saturated fat: 0g,

Cholesterol: 30mg, Sodium: 303mg, Potassium: 481mg,
Carbohydrates: 15.67g, Fiber: 3g, Sugar: 1g, Protein: 1.6g

26. Sautéed Garlic Green Beans

Preparation Time: 10 minutes

Cooking Time: 10 minutes

Servings: 10

Ingredients:

3 lb. green beans, trim med

2 tablespoons olive oil

8 cloves garlic, crushed and minced

½ cup tomato, diced

12 oz. mushrooms

Salt and pepper to taste

Direction

Boil a pot of over.

Add the beans and cook only for 5 minutes.

Drain and remove the water. Pour oil to the pot. Cook the garlic, tomato and mushrooms for 5 minutes.   Season with salt and pepper.

Nutrition: Calories: 74, Total fat: 3.1g, Saturated fat: 0.5g

Sodium: 185mg, Potassium: 438mg, Carbohydrates: 11g, Fiber: 3.6g, Sugar: 5g, Protein: 3.3g

27. Brown Rice Pilaf

Preparation Time: 15 minutes

Cooking Time: 10 minutes

Servings: 5

Ingredients:

2 ½ cups chicken broth

½ cup wild rice

2/3 cup brown rice

2 scallions, chopped

Pepper to taste

Direction

Mix all the ingredients except the brown rice in a pot.

Bring to a boil and then simmer for 10 minutes.

Add the brown rice.   Stir.

Simmer for 30 minutes.

Fluff with a fork before serving.

Nutrition: Calories: 174, Total fat: 1g, Saturated fat: 0.2g, Sodium: 265mg, Potassium: 248mg, Carbohydrates: 35.4g, Fiber: 2.6g

Chapter 8: Dinner

---

28. **Green Curry Tofu**

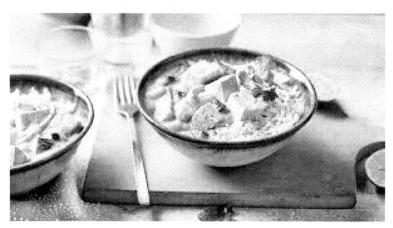

Preparation time: 10 minutes

Cooking time: 15 minutes

Servings: 1

Ingredients:

Lime Juice (1 T.)

Tamari Sauce (1 T.)

Water Chestnuts (8 Oz.)

Green Beans (1 C.)

Salt (.50 t.)

Vegetable Broth (.50 C.)

Coconut Milk (14 Oz.)

Chickpeas (1 C.)

Green Curry Paste (3 T.)

Frozen Edamame (1 C.)

Garlic Cloves (2)

Ginger (1 inch)

Olive Oil (1 t.)

Diced Onion (1)

Extra-firm Tofu (8 Oz.)

Brown Basmati Rice (1 C.)

Directions:

To start, you will want to cook your rice according to the directions on the package. You can do this in a rice cooker or simply on top of the stove.

Next, you will want to prepare your tofu. You can remove the tofu from the package and set it on a plate. Once in place, set another plate on top and something heavy so you can begin to drain the tofu. Once the tofu is prepared, cut it into half inch cubes.

Next, take a medium-sized pan and place it over medium heat. As the pan heats up, go ahead and place your olive oil. When the olive oil begins to sizzle, add your onions and cook until they turn a nice translucent color. Typically, this process will take about five minutes. When your onions are ready, add in the garlic and ginger. With these in place, cook the ingredients for another two to three minutes.

Once the last step is done, add in your curry paste and edamame. Cook these two ingredients until the edamame is no longer frozen.

With these ready, you will now add in the cubed tofu, chickpeas, vegetable broth, coconut milk, and the salt. When everything is in place, you will want to bring the pot to a simmer. Add in the water chestnuts and green beans next and cook for a total of five minutes.

When all the ingredients are cooked through, you can remove the pan from the heat and divide your meal into bowls. For extra flavor, try stirring in tamari, lime juice, or soy sauce. This recipe is excellent served over rice or any other side dish!

Nutrition: Calories: 760, Protein: 23g, Fat: 38g, Carbs: 89g, Fibers: 9g

29. African Peanut Protein Stew

Preparation time: 10 minutes

Cooking time: 30 minutes

Servings: 4

Ingredients:

Basmati Rice (1 Package)

Roasted Peanuts (.25 C.)

Baby Spinach (2 C.)

Chickpeas (15 Oz.)

Chili Powder (1.50 t.)

Vegetable Broth (4 C.)

Natural Peanut Butter (.33 C.)

Pepper (.25 t.)

Salt (.25 t.)

Diced Tomatoes (28 Oz.)

Chopped Sweet Potato (1)

Diced Jalapeno (1)

Diced Red Pepper (1)

Sweet Onion (1)

Olive Oil (1 t.)

Directions:

First, you will want to cook your onion. You will do this by heating olive oil in a large saucepan over medium heat. Once the olive oil is sizzling, add in the onion and cook for five minutes or so. The onion will turn translucent when it is cooked through.

With the onion done, you will now add in the canned tomatoes, diced sweet potato, jalapeno, and bell peppers. Simmer all these ingredients over a medium to high heat for about five minutes. If desired, you can season these vegetables with salt and pepper.

As the vegetables cook, you will want to make your sauce. You will do this by taking a bowl and mix together one cup of vegetable broth with the peanut butter. Be sure to mix well, so there are no clumps. Once this is done, pour the sauce into the saucepan along with three more cups of vegetable broth. At this point, you will want to season the dish with cayenne and chili powder.

Next, cover your pan and reduce to a lower heat. Go ahead and allow these ingredients to simmer for about ten to twenty minutes. At the end of this time, the sweet potato should be nice and tender.

Last, you will want to add in the spinach and chickpeas. Give everything a good stir to mix. You will want to cook this dish until the spinach begins to wilt. Once again, you can add salt and pepper as needed.

Finally, serve your dish over rice, garnish with peanuts, and enjoy!

Nutrition: Calories: 440, Protein: 16g, Fat: 13g, Carbs: 69g, Fibers: 12g

30. Split Pea and Cauliflower Stew

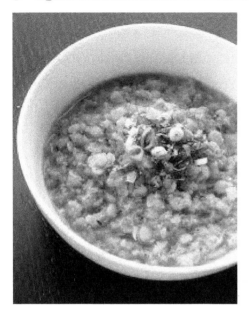

Preparation time: 10 minutes

Cooking time: 60 minutes

Servings: 4

Ingredients:

Green Onions (.25 C.)

Chopped Cilantro (.25 C.)

Salt (1.50 t.)

Garam Masala (1 t.)

Apple Cider Vinegar (2 t.)

Light Coconut Milk (15 Oz.)

Vegetable Broth (2 C.)

Ground Turmeric (1 t.)

Curry Powder (3 t.)

Minced Garlic (6)

Chopped Carrots (2)

Chopped Onion (1)

Cumin Seeds (1 t.)

Mustard Seeds (1 t.)

Spinach Leaves (3 C.)

Chopped Cauliflower (1)

Cooked Split Peas (2 C.)

Directions:

Before you begin cooking this recipe, you will want to prepare your split peas according to the directions on their package.

Once your split peas are cooked, you will want to preheat your oven to 375 degrees. Once warm, place your chopped cauliflower pieces onto a baking sheet and pop it into the oven for ten to fifteen minutes. By the end, the cauliflower should be tender and slightly brown.

Next, you will want to place a large pot on your stove and turn the heat to medium. As the pot heats up, add in the oil, cumin seeds, and mustard seeds. Within sixty seconds, the seeds will begin popping. You will want to make sure you are stirring these ingredients frequently, so they do not burn.

Now that the seeds and oil are warm, you can add in your onion, garlic, ginger, and chopped carrots. Cook these for five minutes or until the carrot and onion are nice and soft. Once they are, you can add in your turmeric and curry powder. Be sure to gently mix everything together so you can evenly coat the vegetables.

After one minute of allowing the vegetables to soak up the spices, you will want to add in the coconut milk, split peas, and vegetable broth. At this point, you will want to lower the heat to low and place a cover over your pot. Allow all the ingredients to simmer for about twenty minutes. As everything cooks, be sure to stir the pot occasionally to make sure nothing sticks to the bottom.

Finally, you will want to stir in the garam masala, apple cider vinegar, and the roasted cauliflower. If needed, you can also add salt as desired. When these ingredients are in place, go ahead and allow the stew to simmer for another ten minutes or so.

As a final touch, feel free to top your stew with green onions and chopped cilantro for extra flavors!

Nutrition: Calories: 700, Protein: 31g, Fat: 31g, Carbs: 84g, Fibers: 34g

31. Black Bean and Pumpkin Chili

Preparation time: 10 minutes

Cooking time: 15 minutes

Servings: 4

Ingredients:

Garbanzo Beans (1 Can)

Black Beans (1 Can)

Vegetable Stock (1 C.)

Tomatoes (1 C.)

Pumpkin Puree (1 C.)

Chopped Onion (1)

Olive Oil (1 T.)

Chili Powder (2 T.)

Cumin Powder (1 T.)

Salt (.25 t.)

Pepper (.25 t.)

Directions:

To begin, you will want to place a large pot over medium heat. At the pot warms up, place your olive oil, garlic, and chopped onion into the bottom. Allow this mixture to cook for about five minutes or until the onion is soft.

At this point, you will now want to add in the garbanzo beans, black beans, vegetable stock, canned tomatoes, and pumpkin. If you do not have any vegetable stock on hand, you can also use water.

With your ingredients in place, add in the half of the chili powder, half of the cumin, and any salt and pepper according to your own taste. Once the spices are in place, give the chili a quick taste and add more as needed.

Now, bring the pot to a boil and stir all the ingredients together to assure the spices are spread evenly throughout your dish.

Last, bring the pot to a simmer and cook everything for about twenty minutes. When the twenty minutes are done, remove the pot from the heat, and enjoy!

Nutrition: Calories: 390, Protein: 19g, Fat: 8g, Carbs: 65g, Fibers: 21g

32. Matcha Tofu Soup

Preparation time: 10 minutes

Cooking time: 55 minutes

Servings: 4

Ingredients:

Vegetable Broth (.5 0 C.)

Extra-firm Tofu (1 Package)

Light Coconut Milk (13.5 Oz.)

Kale (5 C.)

Garlic Powder (.25 t.)

Smoked Paprika (.25 t)

Ground Black Pepper (.25 t.)

Mirin (1 t.)

Soy Sauce (2 T.)

Cilantro (1 C.)

Matcha Powder (2 t.)

Vegetable Broth (4 C.)

Ground Black Pepper (.25 t.)

Cayenne Pepper (.25 t.)

Garlic (1 t.)

Minced Garlic (3)

Chopped Potato (1)

Chopped Onion (1)

Directions:

To start, you will want to place a large pot over medium heat. As the pot warms up, add a splash of vegetable broth to the bottom and begin to cook the chopped potato and onion. Typically, it will take eight to ten minutes until they are nice and soft. When the vegetables are ready, you can then add in the black pepper, cayenne pepper, ginger, and garlic. Sauté these ingredients for another minute.

When these vegetables are prepared, you can add in the kale and cook for a few more minutes. Once the kale begins to wilt, stir in the rest of the vegetable broth and bring your soup to a boil. Once boiling, reduce the heat, cover the pot, and simmer all the ingredients for thirty minutes. After fifteen minutes, remove the top so you can stir in the matcha and cilantro.

Once the thirty minutes are done, remove the pot from the heat and allow the soup to cool for a little. Once cool, place the mixture into a blender and gently stir in the coconut milk.

Blend the soup on high until you reach a silky and smooth consistency for the soup.

Finally, cook your tofu according to your own preference. Be sure to chop the tofu into cubes and brown on all sides. Once cooked, place the tofu in your soup and enjoy!

Nutrition: Calories: 450, Protein: 20g, Fat: 32g, Carbs: 27g, Fibers: 7g

33. Baked Spicy Tofu Sandwich

Preparation time: 10 minutes

Cooking time: 45 minutes

Servings: 4

Ingredients:

Whole Grain Bread (8)

Maple Syrup (1 T.)

White Miso Paste (1 T.)

Tomato Paste (1 T.)

Liquid Smoke (1 Dash)

Soy Sauce (1 T.)

Cumin (1 t.)

Paprika (.50 t.)

Chipotles in Adobo Sauce (1 t.)

Vegetable Broth (1 C.)

Tofu (16 Oz.)

Tomato (1)

Chopped Red Onion (.25 C.)

Tabasco (1 Dash)

Lime (1)

Cumin (.25 t.)

Chili Powder (.25 t.)

Coriander (.25 t.)

Cilantro (.25 C.)

Avocado (1)

Ground Black Pepper (.25 t.)

Garlic (2)

Lime (.50)

Directions:

To prepare for this recipe, you will want to prep your tofu the night before. To start, you will want to press the tofu for a few hours. Once this is done, cut the tofu into eight slices and then place them in the freezer.

When you are ready, it is time to make the marinade for the tofu. To do this, take a bowl and mix together the vegetable broth, tomato paste, maple syrup, and all the spices from the list above. Be sure to stir everything together to get the spices spread through the vegetable broth. Once it is mixed, add in your thawed slices of tofu, and soak them for a few hours.

Once the tofu is marinated, heat your oven to 425 degrees. When the oven is warm, place the tofu on a baking sheet and place in the oven for twenty minutes. At the end of this time, the tofu should be nice and crispy on the top and edges.

When your tofu is cooked to your liking, layer it on your bread slices with your favorite toppings. This sandwich can be enjoyed cold or warm!

Nutrition: Calories: 390, Protein: 21g, Fat: 16g, Carbs: 49g

Fibers: 11g

34. Vegetable Stir-Fry

Preparation time: 10 minutes

Cooking time: 45 minutes

Servings: Three

Ingredients:

Zucchini (.50)

Red Bell Pepper (.50)

Broccoli (.50)

Red Cabbage (1 C.)

Brown Rice (.50 C.)

Tamari Sauce (2 T.)

Red Chili Pepper (1)

Fresh Parsley (.25 t.)

Garlic (4)

Olive Oil (2 T.)

Optional: Sesame Seeds

Directions:

To begin, you will want to cook your brown rice according to the directions that are placed on the package. Once this step is done, place the brown rice in a bowl and put it to the side.

Next, you will want to take a frying pan and place some water in the bottom. Bring the pan over medium heat and then add in your chopped vegetables. Once in place, cook the vegetables for five minutes or until they are tender.

When the vegetables are cooked through, you will then want to add in the parsley, cayenne powder, and the garlic. You will want to cook this mixture for a minute or so. Be sure you stir the ingredients so that nothing sticks to the bottom of your pan.

Now, add in the rice and tamari to your pan. You will cook this mixture for a few more minutes or until everything is warmed through.

For extra flavor, try adding sesame seeds before you enjoy your lunch! If you have any leftovers, you can keep this stir-fry in a sealed container for about five days in your fridge.

Nutrition: Calories: 280, Protein: 10g, Fat: 12g, Carbs: 38g, Fibers: 6g

35. Kale Protein Bowl

Preparation time: 10 minutes

Cooking time: 50 minutes

Servings: Two

Ingredients:

Water (.75 C.)

Maple Syrup (1 t.)

Turmeric (2 t.)

Ground Ginger (.50 t.)

Ground Ginger (.50 t.)

Coconut Aminos (2 T.)

Lime Juice (2 T.)

Tahini (.50 C.)

Hemp Seeds (.25 C.)

Tempeh (4 Oz.)

Broccoli (2 C.)

Kale (3 C.)

Minced Garlic (1)

Coconut Oil (1 T.)

Quinoa (1 C.)

Directions:

Before you put together your bowl, you will want to make your quinoa. Place your quinoa with two cups of water into a pot. Once in place, bring the pot to a boil and reduce the heat. Allow the quinoa to simmer for fifteen minutes or until all the water in the pot is gone. In the end, the quinoa will be nice and fluffy.

Once your quinoa is cooked, take a small saucepan and begin to melt the coconut oil. When the oil begins to sizzle, place your red onion, tempeh, broccoli, kale, and garlic. Cook everything together for about five minutes. By the end, the vegetables should be cooked through and tender.

Now, portion the quinoa into two to three bowls. Once in place, you can top the quinoa off with your cooked vegetables. For extra flavor, drizzle tahini over the top and sprinkle raw hemp seeds. Enjoy!

Nutrition: Calories: 920, Protein: 38g, Fat: 48g, Carbs: 95g, Fibers: 16g

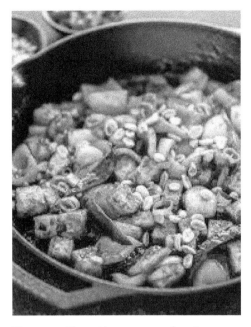

Preparation time: 10 minutes

Cooking time: 40 minutes

Servings: 4

Ingredients:

Water (1 T.)

Sesame Oil (1 t.)

Black Vinegar (2 t.)

Cornstarch (1 t.)

Sugar (2 t.)

Dark Soy Sauce (2 t.)

Light Soy Sauce (1 T.)

Scallions (5)

Sliced Root Ginger (1 In.)

Minced Garlic (3)

Sliced Red Pepper (1)

Sliced Green Pepper (1)

Cooking Oil (3 T.)

Extra-firm Tofu (1 Lb.)

Directions:

Much like with any tofu you cook, you are going to want to make sure you have pressed all the liquid out. Please take the time to press your tofu before you begin cooking, this will leave you with the best results. Once drained, you can cut your tofu into small cubes. At this point, you will also want to cut your green and red pepper into small pieces as well.

Next, you will be making the sauce. You can do this by taking a small bowl and mix the sugar, water, vinegar, cornstarch, garlic, green onion, ginger, salt, and both soy sauces. Be sure to mix everything together well to blend the flavors together.

Next, you will want to take a skillet and place it over medium heat. As the pan warms up, add in three tablespoons of your oil and then gently place the tofu cubes. You will cook the tofu until it becomes a nice golden-brown color on all sides. Once your tofu is cooked, add in the peppers and cook them for another five minutes or so. By the end, the pepper will be nice and tender.

Finally, you will gently pour in the sauce you made earlier. Be sure to stir the ingredients well, so the tofu becomes well coated. Cook this dish over medium heat for another five minutes or so to allow the sauce to begin to thicken. Mix everything well and serve over noodles or steamed rice.

Nutrition: Calories: 300, Protein: 20g, Fat: 22g, Carbs: 13g, Fibers: 5g

37. Black Bean Meatloaf

Preparation time: 10 minutes

Cooking time: 50 minutes

Servings: 4

Ingredients:

Chopped Red Bell Pepper (1)

Quick Oats (1.50 C.)

Black Beans (2 Cans)

Ketchup (3 T.)

Cumin (1 t.)

Liquid Aminos (1 T.)

Minced Garlic (1)

Minced Onion (1)

Chopped Carrot (1)

Black Pepper (.25 t.)

Directions:

First, you will want to heat your oven to 350 degrees. While the oven warms up, you can begin preparing your dinner.

Over medium heat place a medium sized pan and begin to sauté your onions. You can use water or oil to complete this step. As the onion turns translucent, add in your carrot pieces, pepper, and the garlic. You will want to cook these ingredients for six to eight minutes. By the end, the carrots and pepper should be nice and soft.

Next, you will want to get out a large bowl. In this bowl, carefully combine the oats, black beans, and all the seasonings from the list above. Once these are in place, add in the vegetables you just cooked and mash everything together. Combine all the ingredients well but not enough to make the mixture mushy. If the ingredients are too hard to form a "dough," add water or moist oats to help hold everything together. When your dough is ready, you can pour it into a lined loaf pan. Once in place, pop the dish into your heated oven for about thirty minutes. By the end, the edges should develop a nice, browned crust. At this point, you will want to remove the dish from the oven and allow it to cool for a bit. This meal is fantastic alone or can be served with your favorite vegetable side!

Nutrition: Calories: 360, Protein: 18g, Fat: 3g, Carbs: 68g, Fibers: 20g

38. Easy Noodle Alfredo

Preparation time: 10 minutes

Cooking time: 56 minutes

Servings: 4

Ingredients:

Green Peas (1 C.)

Vegan Parmesan Cheese (.25 C.)

Garlic Powder (.50 t.)

Nutritional Yeast (6 T.)

Pepper (.25 t.)

Salt (.25 t.)

Unsweetened Almond Milk (2 C.)

All Purpose Flour (2 T.)

Minced Garlic (4)

Olive Oil (3 T.)

Linguini (10 Oz.)

<u>Directions:</u>

First things first—you will want to cook your linguini. Once this step is complete, drain the water and set the cooked pasta to the side for now.

Next, you will take a large skillet and place it over medium heat. As the pan warms up, carefully add in your garlic and olive oil. You will want to stir these to assure nothing burns to the bottom of your pan.

When you begin to smell the garlic, turn the heat down a tad. Once this is done, add in the flour and cook for about a minute in the olive oil alone. Next, you will add in the almond milk a little bit at a time. Be sure to whisk the ingredients together to help avoid forming clumps in your sauce. Go ahead and cook this sauce for another two minutes or so.

Once your sauce is done, remove from the heat and allow it to cool for a minute or so. When it is safe to handle, transfer the liquid into a blender. When it is in place, add in the garlic, nutritional yeast, vegan parmesan cheese, pepper, and salt according to your taste. Go ahead and blend the mixture on high until you create a nice smooth and creamy sauce. Feel free to adjust your seasonings as you go.

Next, you will want to return the sauce to your pan and place it over medium heat until it begins to bubble. Once the bubbles form, turn the heat to low and allow the sauce to thicken.

Remember to stir your dish frequently to avoid it burning to the bottom.

As you stir the sauce, add more milk if it is too thick. If the sauce is too thin, remove some liquid and add in some extra flour. When the sauce is ready, add it to your pasta and top with cooked peas. For extra flavor, try serving your meal with extra parmesan cheese or even red pepper flakes.

Nutrition: Calories: 470, Protein: 23g, Fat: 7g, Carbs: 82g, Fibers: 10g

39. Hot Potato Curry

Preparation time: 10 minutes

Cooking time: 78 minutes

Servings: Six

Ingredients:

Coconut Milk (14 Oz.)

Peas (15 Oz)

Garbanzo Beans (15 Oz.)

Diced Tomatoes (14.5 Oz.)

Salt (2 t.)

Minced Ginger Root (1)

Garam Masala (4 t.)

Curry Powder (4 t.)

Cayenne Pepper (1.50 t.)

Ground Cumin (2 t.)

Minced Garlic (3)

Diced Yellow Onion (1)

Vegetable Oil (2 T.)

Cubed Potatoes (4)

Directions:

To start, you will want to cook your potatoes. All you need to do is bring a pot of water over high heat until the water begins to boil. When the water begins to boil, reduce the heat and place a cover over the pot. Simmer the potatoes in the water for about fifteen minutes and then drain the water.

As the potatoes are cooking, you will want to bring a large skillet over medium heat. As the pan begins to warm up, place your vegetable oil and onion. Cook the onion for five minutes or until it becomes soft. Now, add in the salt, ginger, garam masala, curry powder, cayenne pepper, cumin, and the garlic. At this point, you will want to cook all these ingredients for two or three minutes.

Once the ingredients are warmed through, add in the cooked potatoes, peas, tomatoes, and the garbanzo beans. When these are all in place, carefully pour in the coconut milk and allow the pan to come to a simmer. Simmer this dish for five to ten minutes and then remove from heat.

This dish is delicious by itself, but feel free to serve with any of your favorite side dishes!

Nutrition:

Calories: 640, Protein: 23g, Fat: 25g, Carbs: 87g, Fibers: 22g

40. Spinach and Red Lentil Masala

Preparation time: 10 minutes

Cooking time: 35 minutes

Servings: 4

Ingredients:

Baby Spinach (2 C.)

Red Lentils (1 C.)

Coconut Milk (15 Oz.)

Salt (1 t.)

Diced Tomatoes (15 Oz.)

Coriander (.25 t.)

Garam Masala (1 t.)

Ground Cumin (1 t.)

Chili Pepper (1)

Minced Ginger (1 In.)

Minced Garlic (2)

Diced Red Onion (1)

Olive Oil (1 T.)

Directions:

To begin, place a large pot over a medium to high heat. As the pot warms up, you can add in your tablespoon of olive oil and the onion. Cook the onion for five minutes or until it becomes soft. Once it does, you can add in the coriander, garam masala, cumin, chili pepper, ginger, and the garlic. When everything is in place, cook the ingredients for an extra two to three minutes. Once the ingredients from the step above are warmed through, you will want to carefully add the tomatoes and season everything with salt according to your taste. If there are any brown bits on the bottom of the pan, be sure to scrape them up and keep stirring everything. As you continue to cook, the liquid should reduce in about five minutes. Next, pour in the coconut milk along with one cup of water. Once in place, turn the heat up to high and bring the pot to a boil. At this point, you can add in the lentils and reduce the heat back to medium or so. Now, cook the lentils for twenty-five to thirty-five minutes. By the end, the lentils should be nice and tender!

Finally, fold in your spinach and cook for an additional five minutes. Once the spinach has wilted, remove the pot from the heat and allow to cool slightly. You can serve this delicious meal over coconut rice or enjoy it by itself.

Nutrition: Calories: 490, Protein: 17g, Fat: 30g, Carbs: 44g, Fibers: 20g

41. Sweet Hawaiian Burger

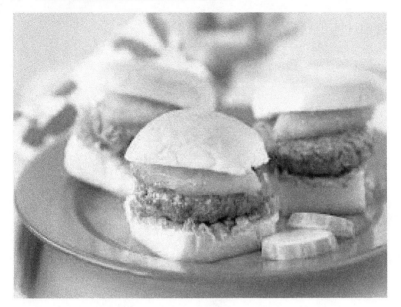

Preparation time: 10 minutes

Cooking time: 15 minutes

Servings: 4

Ingredients:

Panko Breadcrumbs (1 C.)

Red Kidney Beans (14 Oz.)

Vegetable Oil (1 T.)

Diced Sweet Potato (1.50 C.)

Minced Garlic (1)

Soy Sauce (2 T.)

Apple Cider Vinegar (3 T.)

Maple Syrup (.50 C.)

Water (.50 C.)

Tomato Paste (.50 C.)

Pineapple Rings (4)

Salt (.25 t.)

Pepper (.25 t.)

Cayenne (.10 t.)

Ground Cumin (1.50 t.)

Burger Buns (4)

Optional: Red Onion, Tomato, Lettuce, Vegan Mayo

Directions:

First, you will want to heat your oven to 400 degrees. As the oven warms up, take your sweet potato and toss it in oil. When this step is complete, place the diced sweet potato pieces in a single layer on a baking sheet. Once this is done, pop the sheet into the oven and cook for about twenty minutes. Halfway through, flip the pieces over to assure the sweet potato cooks all the way through. When this is done, remove the sheet from the oven and allow the sweet potato to cool down slightly.

Next, you will want to get out your food processor. When you are ready, add in the beans, sweet potatoes, breadcrumbs, cayenne, cumin, soy sauce, garlic, and onion pieces. Once in place, begin to pulse the ingredients together until you have a finely chopped mixture. As you do this, season the "dough" with pepper and salt as desired. Now, shape the dough into four patties.

When your patties are formed, begin to heat a large skillet over medium heat. As the pan warms up, place your oil and then grill each side of your patties. Typically, this will take five to six minutes on each side. You will know the burger is cooked through when it is browned on each side.

All you need to do now is assemble your burger! If you want, try baking the pineapple rings—three minutes on each side should do the trick! Top your burger with lettuce, tomato, and vegan mayo for some extra flavor.

Nutrition: Calories: 460, Protein: 15g, Fat: 12g, Carbs: 80g, Fibers: 6g

Chapter 9: Sauces

42. <u>Lemon Wine Sauce</u>

Preparation Time: 15 minutes

Cooking Time: 10 minutes

Servings: 8

Ingredients:

1 tablespoon olive oil

1 shallot, minced

3 tablespoons freshly squeezed lemon juice

¼ cup dry white wine

½ teaspoon lemon zest

1 tablespoon parsley, chopped

1 tablespoon capers, chopped

1 cup chicken broth

Salt and pepper to taste

1 tablespoon cornstarch

2 tablespoons butter

Direction:

Pour the oil into a pan over medium heat.

Cook the shallot for 1 minute.

Pour in the lemon juice and wine.

Stir in the zest.

Bring to a boil.

Simmer for 3 to 5 minutes.

Add the parsley, capers and broth.

Season with salt and pepper.

Cook for 5 minutes.

Mix the cornstarch and water.

Stir the cornstarch mixture into the sauce.

Add the butter and cook until melted.

Refrigerate for up to 3 days.

Nutrition: Calories: 46, Total fat: 3.2g, Saturated fat: 1.1g, Cholesterol: 4mg, Sodium: 116mg, Potassium: 51mg, Carbohydrates: 2.8g, Fiber: 0.1g, Sugar: 1g, Protein: 0.6g

43. Pumpkin Sauce

Preparation time: 5 minutes

Cooking time: 2 minutes

Servings: 6

30ml olive oil

3 cloves garlic, minced

15g cornstarch

400g pumpkin puree

300ml soy milk

45g nutritional yeast

Direction:

Heat olive oil in a saucepan.

Add garlic and cook for 2 minutes, over medium-high heat.

Add cornstarch and stir to combine. Whisk in soy milk and bring to a boil. Reduce heat and stir in the pumpkin. Simmer for 2 minutes. Stir in nutritional yeast.

Remove from heat and serve.

Nutrition: Calories 208, Total Fat 9.8g, Total Carbohydrate 20.8g, Dietary Fiber 4.7g, Total Sugars 6.7g, Protein 10.9g

44. Spicy Chickpeas

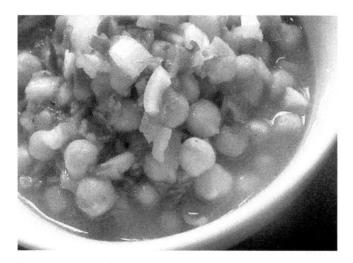

Preparation time: 5 minutes

Cooking time: 10 minutes

Servings: 4

Ingredients:

400g chickpeas, rinsed, drained

45ml olive oil

1 onion, cut in half

3 cloves garlic

350ml chickpea water

3 sprigs rosemary, chopped

½ teaspoon red pepper flakes

Salt and pepper, to taste

Direction:

Heat olive oil in a saucepan.

Add onion and cook 5 minutes.

Add garlic and cook 2 minutes, over medium heat.

Add chickpeas, chickpea water, rosemary, and red pepper flakes.

Simmer for 10 minutes.

Transfer the mixture to a food blender.

Blend on high until smooth.

Serve with pasta.

Nutrition: Calories 394, Total Fat 17.3g, Total Carbohydrate 67.2g, Dietary Fiber 18.9g, Total Sugars 12g, Protein 21.2g.

45. Creamy Tofu Sauce

Preparation time: 5 minutes

Servings: 2

Ingredients:

350g silken tofu

40ml soy milk

2 clove garlic

¼ teaspoon paprika

¼ teaspoon cayenne

1 tablespoon dried parsley

1 tablespoon dried basil

Salt and pepper, to taste

Direction:

Toss all ingredients into a food blender.

Blend on high until smooth.

Serve with pasta or rice.

Nutrition: Calories 127, Total Fat 5.2g,
Total Carbohydrate 6.9g, Dietary Fiber 0.6g, Total Sugars
3.2g, Protein 13.1g

46. Spinach Sauce

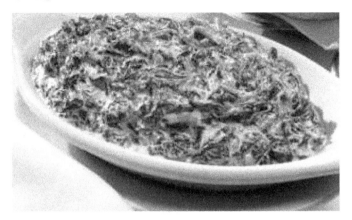

Preparation time: 5 minutes

Cooking time: 3 minutes

Servings: 2

Ingredients:

150g fresh spinach

20g fresh basil

240ml soy milk

5g nutritional yeast

15g cornstarch

2 cloves garlic

½ teaspoon onion powder

Salt and pepper, to taste

1 pinch nutmeg

Direction:

Place all ingredients in a food blender.

Blend on high until smooth.

Transfer to a saucepot.

Bring to a simmer. Cook over medium heat for 3 minutes.

Serve warm.

Nutrition: Calories 127, Total Fat 2.7g, Total Carbohydrate 19.6g, Dietary Fiber 3.2g, Total Sugars 5.3g, Protein 7.7g

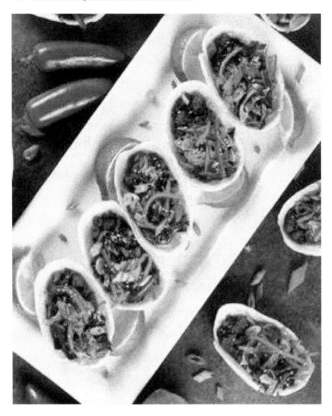

Preparation time: 5 minutes

Cooking time: 8 minutes

Servings: 2

Ingredients:

15ml olive oil

½ small onion, diced

2 cloves garlic, minced

400g can red kidney beans, rinsed, drained

30ml balsamic vinegar

30g tomato paste

½ teaspoon cayenne pepper

½ teaspoon smoked paprika

Salt, to taste

Direction:

Heat olive oil in a skillet.

Add onion and cook 5 minutes, over medium-high heat.

Add garlic and cook 2 minutes.

Toss in the beans, balsamic vinegar, tomato paste, and spices.

Cook 1 minute.

Transfer the mixture to a food blender.   Blend on high until smooth.

Serve with pasta, falafel, or tacos.

Nutrition: Calories 342, Total Fat 8.2g,
Total Carbohydrate 51.2g, Dietary Fiber 15.9g,
Total Sugars 3.3g, Protein 18.4g

48. Hemp Alfredo Sauce

Preparation time: 5 minutes

Servings: 4

Ingredients:

125g raw cashews, soaked in water for 2 hours

80g raw hemp seeds

115ml soy milk

10g nutritional yeast

15ml lemon juice

2 cloves garlic, minced

Salt, to taste

Direction:

Drain the cashews and place in a food processor.

Add the remaining ingredients and process on high until smooth.

Serve with pasta or soba noodles.

Nutrition:

Calories 319, Total Fat 23.2g, Total Carbohydrate 17g, Dietary Fiber 1.7g, Total Sugars 3.5g, Protein 13.5g

49. Vegan Cheese Sauce

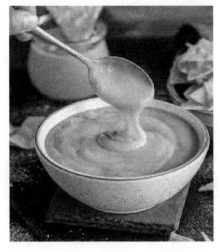

Preparation time: 10 minutes

Cooking time: 15 minutes

Servings: 6

Ingredients:

450g sweet potatoes, peeled, cubed

150g grated carrots

100g raw cashews, soaked in water 2 hours, drained

65g red lentils, picked, rinsed

30g rolled oats

20g nutritional yeast

30g miso paste

15ml lemon juice

950ml water

10g garlic powder

Salt, to taste

Direction:

Combine water, potatoes, carrots, cashews, lentils, and oats in a saucepot.

Bring to a boil.

Reduce heat and simmer 15 minutes.

Strain through a fine-mesh sieve. Reserve some of the cooking liquid if you need to thin the sauce.

Transfer the cooked ingredients into a food blender.

Add nutritional yeast, miso paste, lemon juice, garlic powder, and season to taste.

Blend until smooth. If needed, add some cooking liquid to thin down the sauce.

Serve with pasta, potatoes, or with poutine.

Nutrition: Calories 278, Total Fat 8.8g, Total Carbohydrate 42.6g, Dietary Fiber 9.2g, Total Sugars 3.5g, Protein 9.5g

50. Pea Cheesy Sauce

Preparation time: 5 minutes

Servings: 2

Ingredients:

160g frozen peas, defrosted

20 leaves basil

30g nutritional yeast

30ml lemon juice

45ml vegetable stock

Salt, to taste

1 clove garlic

Direction:

Combine all ingredients, except the vegetable stock in a food blender. Blend until smooth.

Gradually add in the vegetable stock, until desired consistency is reached.

Serve.

Nutrition: Calories 123, Total Fat 1.5g, Total Carbohydrate 18.5g, Dietary Fiber 8.2g, Total Sugars 4.2g, Protein 11.7g

51. Orange & Honey Sauce

Preparation Time: 15 minutes

Cooking Time: 15 minutes

Servings: 8

Ingredients:

1 tablespoon olive oil

¼ cup chopped shallot

¼ cup freshly squeezed orange juice

½ teaspoon orange zest

1 cup champagne

1 tablespoon honey

Salt and pepper to taste

¼ teaspoon ground coriander

1 tablespoon cornstarch

2 tablespoons dry white wine

1 tablespoon butter

Direction:

Pour the oil into a pan over medium heat.

Cook the shallot for 1 minute.

Stir in the orange juice, orange zest, champagne, honey, salt, pepper and coriander.

Bring to a boil.

Cook for 10 minutes.

In a bowl, mix the cornstarch and wine.

Add this mixture to the pan.

Stir in butter and cook until melted.

Refrigerate for up to 3 days.

Nutrition: Calories: 83, Total fat: 3.2g, Saturated fat: 1.1g, Cholesterol: 4mg, Sodium: 74mg, Potassium: 35mg, Carbohydrates: 5.5g, Fiber: 0.1g, Sugar: 3g, Protein: 0.4g

52. Butternut Squash Sauce

Preparation Time: 10 minutes

Cooking Time: 13 minutes

Servings: 12

Ingredients:

2 cups water

½ cup cashew, chopped

2 tablespoons olive oil

2 sweet onions, diced

2 tablespoons garlic, minced

½ teaspoon salt

¼ cup dry white wine

¾ teaspoon dried oregano

1 cup butternut squash puree

⅛ teaspoon ground nutmeg

Pepper to taste

Direction

Blend cashews and water in a food processor until smooth. Set aside.

Pour the oil into a pan over medium heat.

Cook the onion and garlic for 3 minutes.

Season with salt.

Reduce heat and cook for another 10 minutes.

Stir in the wine and oregano.

Add the squash puree, nutmeg and cashew.

Cook for 3 minutes.

Refrigerate for up to 3 days.

Nutrition: Calories: 102, Total fat: 5.3g, Saturated fat: 0.9g, Sodium: 184mg, Potassium: 216mg, Carbohydrates: 10.9g, Fiber: 2.1g, Sugar: 4g, Protein: 1.8g

Preparation Time: 15 minutes

Cooking Time: 10 minutes

Servings: 10

Ingredients:

1 tablespoon olive oil

1 shallot, minced

1 cup dry red wine

1 tablespoon sugar

¼ cup frozen cranberries

¼ cup dried cranberries

Salt and pepper to taste

1 teaspoon fresh sage, chopped

1 tablespoon cornstarch

1 tablespoon butter

Direction:

Pour the oil into a pan over medium heat.

Cook the shallot for 1 minute.

Add the wine, sugar, cranberries, salt, pepper and sage.

Bring to a boil.

Simmer for 10 minutes.

Mix the cornstarch and butter.

Add to the sauce.

Simmer for 2 minutes.

Refrigerate for up to 3 days.

Nutrition: Calories: 79, Total fat: 2.6g, Saturated fat: 0.9g, Cholesterol: 3mg, Sodium: 61mg, Potassium: 64mg, Carbohydrates: 7.3g, Fiber: 0.4g, Sugar: 5g, Protein: 0.2g

Chapter 10: Vegan Cheese

54. **Vegan Vegetable Cheese Sauce**

Preparation Time: 10 minutes

Cooking Time: 10 minutes

Servings: 4

Ingredients:

2 pcs. small potatoes, peeled and sliced into ¼-inch pieces

1 pc. carrot, peeled and sliced into ¼-inch pieces

2 tbsp. nutritional yeast

2 tbsp. extra-virgin olive oil

Half a lemon's juice

A pinch of garlic salt and cayenne pepper powder

Minced roasted red peppers, cayenne peppers, or jalapeño (optional)

Directions:

Put the potatoes and carrots in a pot. Pour in hot water and cook under low heat.

Once the vegetables are cooked, drain the water.

Put the cooked vegetables in a blender with all the other ingredients. You can also add in the optional ingredients at this point.

Blend all the ingredients together until it's smooth.

Transfer the sauce to a serving dish. You can enjoy it with some nachos or steamed broccoli.

Nutrition: Calories: 360, Protein: 18g, Fat: 3g, Carbs: 68g, Fibers: 20g

55. Easy Nut-Free Vegan Cheese Sauce

Preparation Time: 10 minutes

Cooking Time: 50 minutes

Servings: 4

 Ingredients:

340 g soft or silken tofu

¼ cup nutritional yeast

½ cup unsweetened soy milk

1 tbsp. white wine vinegar

2 tsp. Dijon mustard

1 ½ tsp. onion powder

1 tsp. salt

½ tsp. garlic powder

¼ tsp. paprika, smoked

Directions:

Combine all the ingredients in a blender. Blend until you get a smooth mixture.

Pour the mixture into a saucepan and warm the cheese over low heat. Constantly stir to avoid burning the cheese.

Put the heated mixture into a serving bowl and enjoy it with other dishes or treats.

Nutrition: Calories: 120, Protein: 8g, Fat: 3g, Carbs: 8g, Fibers: 10g

56. White Beans Vegan Cheese Sauce

Preparation Time: 10 minutes

Cooking Time: 10 minutes

Servings: 4

Ingredients:

1 cup white beans, cooked

½ cup plant-based milk of your choice

5 tbsp. nutritional yeast

½ tsp. salt

1/8 tsp. garlic powder

½ tsp apple cider or white vinegar

2 tsp. olive oil

A pinch of dried herbs and spices you prefer (optional)

Directions:

Blend all the ingredients in a blender or food processor until smooth.

Pour the pureed mixture into a pot over low heat and stir occasionally. You can add more milk if the cheese is too thick for you.

Instead of doing Step 2, you can transfer the puree into an instant pot. Set the heat to manual and let it heat up for about 5 minutes.

Transfer it to a serving dish or use it for other dishes.

Nutrition: Calories: 234, Protein: 18g, Fat: 3g, Carbs: 34g, Fibers: 20g

Preparation Time: 10 minutes

Cooking Time: 15 minutes

Servings: 4

Ingredients:

1 cup raw cashews, soaked for 12 hours

1 cup sweet potato, pureed

½ cup vegetable broth

1 tsp. apple cider vinegar

¼ cup nutritional yeast

½ tsp. salt

Directions:

Put all the ingredients in a blender or food processor. Blend until you get a smooth puree.

If the mixture seems too thick, add a bit more vegetable broth. Add in 1 tablespoon at a time until it reaches the consistency you desire.

Transfer the cheese to a bowl and use it as you like.

Nutrition: Calories: 236, Protein: 18g, Fat: 3g, Carbs: 68g, Fibers: 20g

58. Simple Firm Vegan Cheese

Preparation Time: 10 minutes

Cooking Time: 10 minutes

Servings: 4

Ingredients:

1 cup cashew or soy milk, or 1 cup water + 1/3 cup soaked cashew

1 cup sweet potato, boiled

1 tbsp. soy sauce

½ tsp. cumin

½ tsp. paprika

1 tsp. salt

2 tbsp. nutritional yeast

2 cloves of garlic or 2 tsp. garlic powder

Half a lemon's juice

2 ½ tbsp. agar-agar powder

1 cup cold water

Directions:

In a blender, combine all the ingredients except for the cold water and agar-agar powder. Blend them all until you get a smooth mixture.

Pour in the water in a small saucepan and add the agar-agar powder.

Mix the water and agar-agar powder well. Then, place the saucepan over low to medium heat.

Continue to mix until the agar-agar powder is completely dissolved. This will take about 5 minutes.

Add the agar-agar mixture in the blender. Blend it well with the pureed mixture.

Pour the mixture into your molds. You can use a ceramic bowl or silicon molds if they're available.

Place the cheese in the refrigerator for about 30 minutes or until the cheese has set.

Remove the cheese from the molds and serve.

Nutrition: Calories: 220, Protein: 10g, Fat: 2g, Carbs: 6g, Fibers: 25g

59. Easy Cashew Vegan Cheese

Preparation Time: 10 minutes

Cooking Time: 20 minutes

Servings: 4

 Ingredients:

½ cup cashews, soaked in hot water for 1 hour and drained

3 tbsp. nutritional yeast

1 tbsp. cider vinegar or lemon juice

1 tbsp. maple syrup

1 ½ tsp. cornstarch

1 ½ tsp. agar-agar powder

½ tsp. salt

Half a clove of garlic

1 cup water, divided into two ½ cups

Preferred herbs and spices (optional)

Directions:

Mix all the ingredients in a blender or food processor except for the agar-agar powder and ½ cup water. Blend for about 1 minute or until you get a creamy texture.

Heat ½ cup water with agar-agar powder in a saucepan.

Add the blended mixture to the saucepan. Bring to a boil while stirring constantly.

Lightly brush your ceramic molds with oil. Then, pour the mixture into the molds.

Refrigerate the cheese for 2 hours or more.

Remove the cheese from the molds and serve.

Nutrition: Calories: 167, Protein: 14g, Fat: 4g, Carbs: 6g, Fibers: 10g

60. Vegan Nut Cheese

Preparation Time: 10 minutes

Cooking Time: 10 minutes

Servings: 4

Ingredients:

½ cup raw cashews, soaked for 3 hours and drained

1/3 cup water

1 tbsp. coconut oil

1 tsp apple cider vinegar

Half a lemon's juice

A pinch of salt

Directions:

In a blender, mix all the ingredients until smooth.

Line ramekins or other molds you have with plastic wrap.

Pour the cheese mixture into the molds.

Refrigerate for at least 2 hours or until the cheese is set. You may also freeze it if you want to speed things up.

Remove the cheese by turning the molds upside-down on a serving dish.

Remove the plastic wrap from the cheese and enjoy.

Nutrition: Calories: 360, Protein: 18g, Fat: 3g, Carbs: 68g, Fibers: 20g

61. Vegan American Cheese

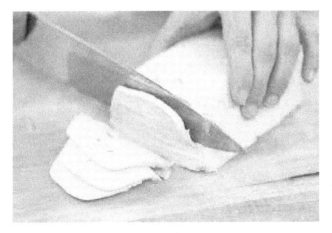

Preparation Time: 10 minutes

Cooking Time: 10 minutes

Servings: 4

Ingredients:

1 cup raw cashews, soaked and drained

¼ cup water

¼ cup lemon juice

1/3 cup nutritional yeast

1 red bell pepper, chopped

2 garlic cloves chopped

2 tbsp. red onion, chopped

1 tsp. yellow mustard

1 tsp. sea salt

½ cup cold water

4 tsp. agar-agar powder

Directions:

In a blender, mix all the ingredients except for the cold water and agar-agar powder. Leave the mixture in the blender.

In a saucepan, mix in cold water and agar-agar powder. Stir for 5 minutes over medium heat and bring it to a boil.

Once it starts to boil, adjust the heat to low and let it simmer while constantly whisking for 8 minutes.

Pour in the agar-agar mixture to the blender and process it again until everything is well-combined.

Pour the mixture into a lined rectangular baking pan that's at least ½ to an inch deep. Only fill halfway if you're using a ½-inch deep pan (quarter-filled for an inch-deep pan).

Refrigerate the cheese for at least 2 hours or until firm.

Cut the cheese into desired sizes and wrap each piece in waxed paper.

Nutrition: Calories: 188, Protein: 18g, Fat: 3g, Carbs: 14g, Fibers: 20g

62. Vegan Cottage Cheese

Preparation Time: 10 minutes

Cooking Time: 5 minutes

Servings: 4

Ingredients:

1 ½ cups firm tofu

1/3 cups silken tofu

1 tbsp. nutritional yeast

1 tsp. lemon juice

1 tsp. apple cider vinegar

½ tsp salt

Directions:

Use a blender to combine all the ingredients except for the firm tofu. Blend until you get a smooth mixture.

Pour the tofu mixture into a medium mixing bowl.

Break the firm tofu into small pieces and place it in the tofu mixture. Mix well and serve.

Nutrition: Calories: 360, Protein: 18g, Fat: 3g, Carbs: 68g, Fibers: 20g

63. Herbs + Garlic Soft Cheese

Preparation Time: 10 minutes

Cooking Time: 20 minutes

Servings: 4

 Ingredients:

2 cups cashews, soaked in cold water and refrigerated for 12 hours

Zest from 1 medium lemon

Juice from 2 medium lemons

¾ cup water

2 garlic cloves, minced (should yield 1 tbsp.)

2 tbsp. nutritional yeast

2 tbsp. olive oil

½ tsp. garlic powder

½ tsp. sea salt

2 tbsp. fresh dill, finely minced

Directions:

After soaking the cashews, drain and put them into a food processor.

Add all the other ingredients except for the fresh dill.

Start grinding and processing the ingredients until you get a smooth and creamy puree. You can taste it and add more ingredients until you get your desired flavor.

Place a colander or a mesh strainer over a mixing bowl. Then, lay down cheesecloth over the colander. Use about two layers.

Scoop the cheese and put it on the cheesecloth. Get all the corners of the cheesecloth and gather them, trapping the cheese inside. Gently twist the top to shape the cheese into a thick disc. Finally, secure it with one or two rubber bands.

Refrigerate the cheese and let it sit for about 6 to 12 hours. The longer you let it set, the better. This is to make sure that all the excess moisture is gone and that your cheese will hold its shape. Unwrap the cheesecloth once ready to serve. Place the cheese on a serving dish. You can reshape it with your hands if needed.

Coat the cheese with chopped fresh dill and add more lemon zest if preferred.

Nutrition: Calories: 178, Protein: 18g, Fat: 3g, Carbs: 20g, Fibers: 11g

64. Vegan Mozzarella Cheese

Preparation Time: 10 minutes

Cooking Time: 15 minutes

Servings: 4

 Ingredients:

1 cup cashews, soaked in cold water and refrigerated for at least 4 hours

¼ cup unsweetened soy milk

1 ¼ cup unsweetened dairy-free yogurt

3 1/3 tbsp. tapioca starch

2 tbsp. lemon juice

2 tbsp. refined coconut oil

2 tsp. nutritional yeast

1 ½ tsp. sea salt

¼ tsp. garlic powder

2 tsp. agar-agar powder

½ cup water

Directions:

In a medium container, create a brine. Fill the container halfway with some filtered water, 5-6 pieces of ice cubes, and a few pinches of sea salt.

Drain the cashews and put it inside a food processor or blender. Also add in the milk, yogurt, tapioca starch, lemon juice, coconut oil, nutritional yeast, sea salt, and garlic powder.

Process or blend them on high for about 2 minutes or until you get a smooth mixture.

Next, add the ½ cup of the filtered water to a medium-sized pot and place it over medium heat.

When the water starts to get hot, whisk in your agar-agar powder. Whisk it well and it should start looking like gel after 3 to 4 minutes.

Once this happens, pour the blended mixture in the pot. Continuously stir using a silicone spatula to avoid your cheese from burning or sticking.

After a few minutes, the cheese will become thicker. Once it becomes thick and stretchy, remove the pan from the heat.

Use an ice cream scooper to shape the mixture into balls. Drop each ball into the brine you made earlier.

After scooping all the mixture, cover the container and put it in the refrigerator. Keep the cheese refrigerated for at least 3 hours before serving.

Nutrition: Calories: 360, Protein: 18g, Fat: 3g, Carbs: 68g, Fibers: 20g

65. Vegan Cotija Cheese

Preparation Time: 10 minutes

Cooking Time: 15 minutes

Servings: 4

 Ingredients:

1 cup almonds, slivered

2 tsp. lemon juice

2 tsp. manzanilla olives brine

A few pinches of salt

Directions:

Put the almonds, salt, lemon juice, and brine in a blender or food processor.

Blend or process the ingredients until they become crumbly in texture. This should take about 4-5 minutes. Taste and add more salt if needed. Also, don't over process the mixture to avoid getting almond butter instead.

Place the mixture into about 2 sheets of cheesecloth. Use these to squeeze out all the liquid from the cheese.

Secure the cheesecloth and put it in the fridge. Keep it refrigerated for about 24 hours.

Open the cheesecloth and transfer the cheese to a container. Crumble the cheese and use as desired.

Nutrition: Calories: 278, Protein: 18g, Fat: 3g, Carbs: 68g, Fibers: 20g

66. Two-Ways Vegan Feta Cheese

Preparation Time: 10 minutes

Cooking Time: 10 minutes

Servings: 4

 Ingredients:

12 oz. (350 g) tofu, extra-firm

½ cup refined coconut oil, melted

3 tbsp. lemon juice

2 tbsp. apple cider vinegar

1 tbsp. nutritional yeast

1 tsp. onion powder

½ tsp. garlic powder

¼ tsp. dill, dried

2 tsp. salt

Directions:

Put all the ingredients in a food processor. But use only a teaspoon of salt.

Process the ingredients until you get a smooth texture. Taste the mixture and add in more salt if needed. Blend it again if you decide to add more salt.

Spreadable Feta You can already serve the feta cheese after processing if you want a spreadable version of this cheese. You may also put the cheese in a container to refrigerate for a few hours. This will make the cheese a bit firmer and easier to put on a cheese board.

Firm and Crumbly Feta If you want your feta cheese to be crumbly, firm, and shaped into cubes, follow these Direction:

Line a rectangular or square-shaped baking dish with parchment paper. Use a pan where you can spread the cheese to be 1-to 2-inch thick.

Spread the cheese into your baking dish. Push down evenly, making sure that there are no air pockets.

Cover and refrigerate the cheese for about 2 hours. This will prevent the coconut oil from separating from your cheese.

While waiting for the cheese, preheat your oven to 200°C or 400 °F.

Remove the cheese from the refrigerator and take off the cover. Bake it for 35 minutes.

Take it out from your oven. Don't worry if the cheese seems bubbly and soft. It will set once it's cooled down.

Let the cheese cool and place in the fridge for at least 4 hours.

Cut the cheese into cubes or crumble before serving or using.

Nutrition: Calories: 360, Protein: 18g, Fat: 3g, Carbs: 68g, Fibers: 20g

Conclusion

I would like to thank you once again for downloading my book, and I hope you enjoyed it. Hopefully, I was able to clarify why it is so important that we have protein in our diet and how you CAN do it as a vegan.

So, do not be afraid of this diet and feel that you are not capable of reaching the lifestyle that you desire! Yes, it may take time but do not be scared to make the transition. With a little effort, research and dedication, you will find that it is much easier to live a healthy vegan lifestyle! Happy reading!

There are going to be many doubters out there in the world—do not let them convince you that your diet is wrong. You are the only person you need to convince that a vegan diet is the best option for you.

You have made the decision to not only better your health but also make the world around you better. At this point, you are saving animals and helping the environment. Your diet choices are beneficial to you and the world around you. Now, you know just how delicious your diet can be. While some look at a vegan diet as restrictive, you know better. As a vegan, you get to have your cake and eat it as well!

Best of luck to you and I hope this book helps you make amazing tasting vegan recipes!

CPSIA information can be obtained
at www.ICGtesting.com
Printed in the USA
BVHW041347020321
601493BV00012B/1060